UNWIN BROTHERS'

LOOKING BACK
SERIES

A series of reminiscences and personal documents from the past
edited by John Fines, M.A.(Cantab.), Ph.D.(Sheffield)

Vol. 2

A YOUNG SURGEON IN WELLINGTON'S ARMY

Compiled by
Leonard W. Woodford, B.A. (Keele)

UNWIN BROTHERS LIMITED
The Gresham Press
OLD WOKING, SURREY, ENGLAND

Printed and published by
UNWIN BROTHERS LIMITED
The Gresham Press
Old Woking, Surrey, GU22 9LH, ENGLAND.

ISBN 0-9502121-8-0

COVER DESIGN: CARTOUCHE, BOLOGNESE SCHOOL, early 17th century. REPRODUCED BY GRACIOUS PERMISSION OF HER MAJESTY THE QUEEN.

FRONT COVER: 'FRENCH WOUNDED ON THE ISLAND OF LOBAU ON THE DANUBE AFTER THE BATTLE OF ESSLING', by C. Meynier. Courtesy of the RADIO TIMES HULTON PICTURE LIBRARY.

BACK COVER: 'STORMING OF ST. SEBASTIAN, August 31st, 1813', by W. Heath.
Courtesy of the NATIONAL ARMY MUSEUM:

Also: 'THE VICTORY OF VITTORIA', by I. M. Wright, 'AN ENSIGN BEARING THE REGIMENTAL COLOURS OF THE IXTH OR E. NORFOLK REGIMENT'.

'LIST OF EXAMINERS 20th APRIL, 1810', by kind permission of the President and Council of the ROYAL COLLEGE OF SURGEONS OF ENGLAND'

NEW VOLUMES OF THE UNWIN BROTHERS' 'LOOKING BACK' SERIES WILL APPEAR AT REGULAR INTERVALS

This series is designed to provide for students and the general reader a personal view of the great events of history. Those who have participated in the past at a high level have left memoirs, but these often tend to be self-centred, and they contain a vision of events only at high class or administrative level. What we often lack is the view of the ordinary private citizen, the man in the street round whom events circulated. Perhaps the man in the street does not see as much as the member of the government but what he does see is more of the reality, the outside of a situation, and the liveliness of memory of the ordinary person is not hampered and constrained by official requirements, by the need to protect colleagues and one's own image.

Vol. 1 is entitled 'A MEMOIR OF AN ENGLISH GOVERNESS IN RUSSIA, 1914–1917'. Mrs Dawe née Dowse participated in Russian life before and during the Revolution on a low level, as a foreign observer, trapped in a situation that seemed remote. Much of the feel of those events that we have to study in the clipped and official tones of those who participated out of desire or need is conveyed in these memoirs in wholly different and more immediate language. For she tells of those days in our tongue, not just in English, but in the language of ordinary interested people.

Vol. 3 is entitled 'LIFE AT SEA, A NINETEENTH CENTURY VOYAGE TO NEW ZEALAND' being the diary of John Grayson a boot-maker who left Navenby station on 18th November, 1875 and arrived in New Zealand on 26th February, 1876 recording numerous events during the months at sea.

JOHN FINES is head of history at Bishop Otter College of Education, Chichester. He received his first degree at Cambridge and later took a PhD at the University of Sheffield. His work takes him into a wide range of schools which experience has aided his preparation of materials for use in history teaching. He has published extensively on educational, medieval and sixteenth century studies.

DRAMATIS PERSONAE

WILLIAM DENT: *I arrived in Colchester a fortnight ago, and was very much suprised to find such a number of Men sick as there is; there are only five Assistants now at this place, two having been sent to Meely Barracks where there is likewise a great number of Sick; each assistant is placed under a separate Surgeon, I am placed under a very nice Man of the name of Hill who is Surgeon to the first Battalion of the fourth Regiment which is come from Spain, and in that Regiment alone there is one hundred and ninety seven Men sick and wounded in the hospital, and half of this number I have to take care of myself.*

HIS FATHER: *By some unaccountable delay I have not been able to send the box till this day, however I hope it will arrive safe; and the Glass, Pipe, and Boot Jack, will meet my Fathers satisfaction.*

HIS COUSIN ANTHONY HARRISON: *When you see* ANTHY *Harrison and his Wife, give my best respects to them, and also the Children; for although he may appear to have acted negligently towards himself, and ungratefully to his friends at home, yet I shall always feel the greatest friendship for his attention to me while at Barnard Castle.*

HIS MOTHER: *I dare not say anything against her smoking, for it has become so habitual that I suppose it would almost destroy her to leave it off; however you may tell her that I hope she makes use of a* cleaner Pipe *than when I last saw her.*

HIS BROTHER KITT: *I hope the Plot of Ground at Lund Hill is gradually improving, I assure you I often think of it, and if I live as long intend to spend my Cottage Days there; Brother* Kitt *it is expected, pays every attention to it, but from his great partially for* Rabbits *and* Ducks, *I have my doubts of the fact.*

HIS BROTHER JOHN: *Had it been John my surprise would have been much less, for he was always famed for an amourous disposition . . . .*

JANE FALLOWFIELD: *I suppose Jane Fallowfield told you about Jack, if she be at Mickleton, be so kind as to remember me to her, but perhaps she has forgot there ever was such a boy as myself.*

LORD WELLINGTON: *We have no late arrivals from Lisbon but I believe both Armies continue in the same position, I think there is little doubt but Lord Wellington will ultimately be driven out of the Country. (17th Feby. 1813) Lord Wellington has joined the Army but there is no symptom of its being collected for some time time yet, in consequence of the number sick.*

THE SCENE: LONDON, COLCHESTER, PORTSMOUTH, GIBRALTAR, VILLA REAL, VILLA NEUVA, SALVATIERRA, SAN SEBASTIAN, ST. JEAN de LUZ, BAYONNE, BIDENT, ST. RHONE, CANADA, GHENT, ST. AMAND, ECOUEIR, ENE, DAYMES, CAMBRAI, GOSPORT, ST. VINCENTS, DOMINICA, GRENADA, TRINIDAD, LONDON.

A Young Surgeon in Wellington's Army

The Letters of William Dent

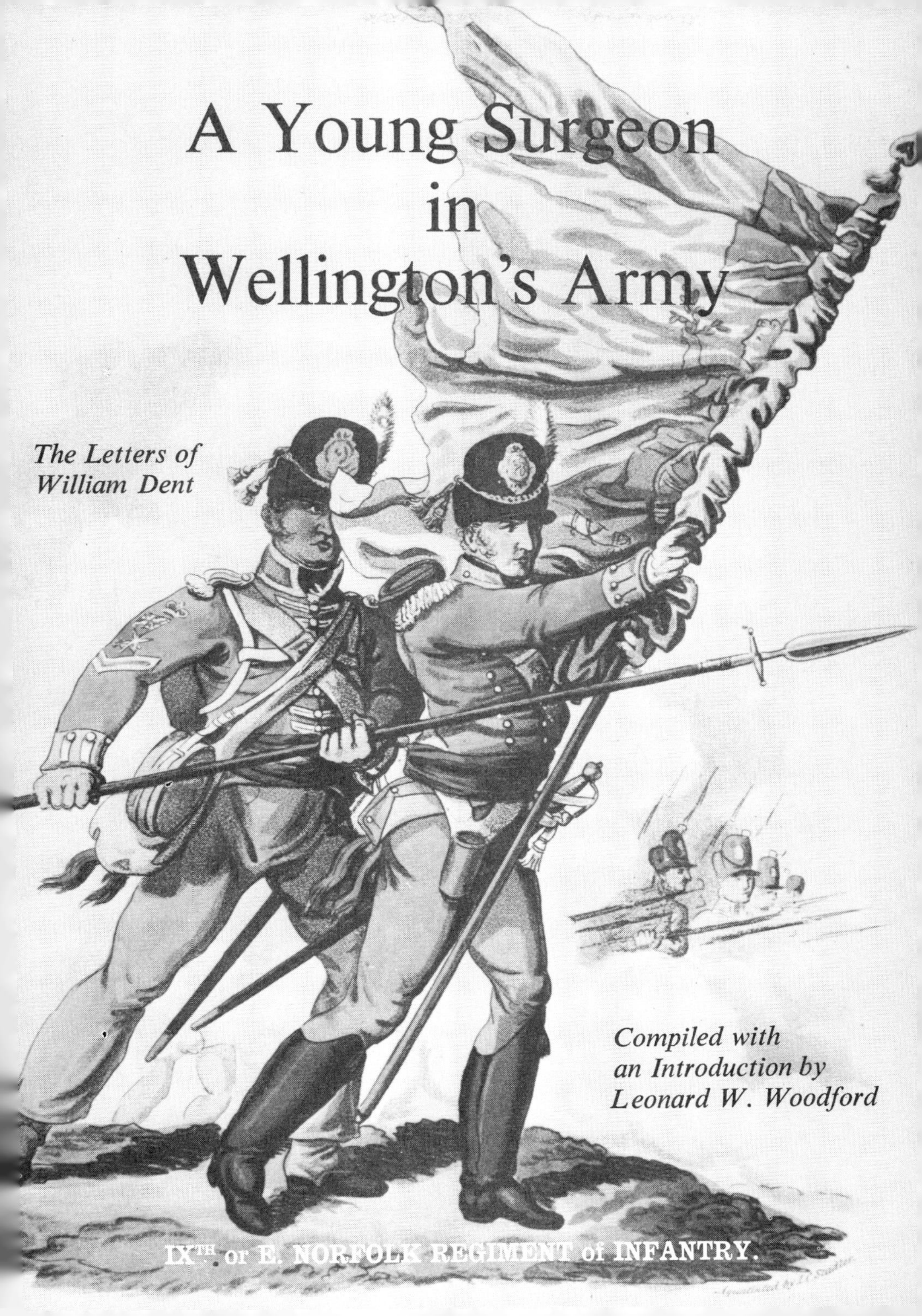

Compiled with an Introduction by Leonard W. Woodford

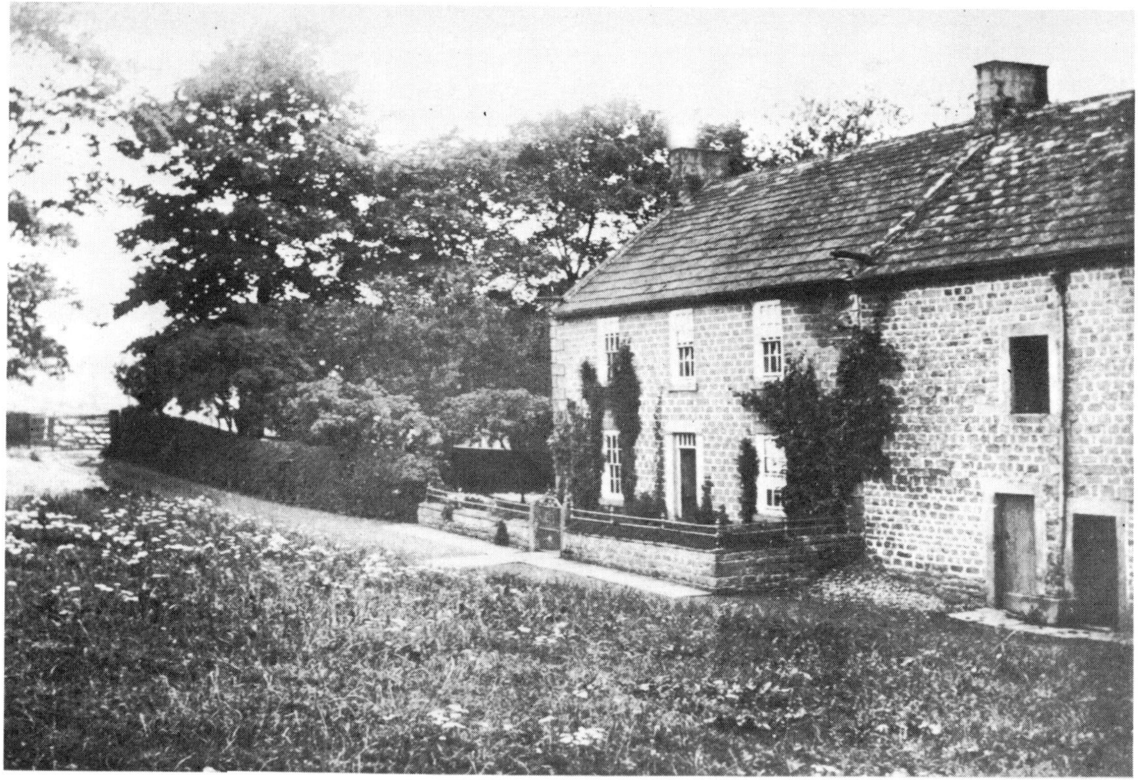

Low Green, William Dent's Birthplace

THE DENT LETTERS—1808–1824

The Dent family are known to have farmed at Mickleton-in-Teesdale on the Durham/Yorkshire border since the 1520s and possibly even earlier. The present generation living there bring to mind the words of composer Edward German when he asked, "Where are the yeomen the yeomen of England?" and the answer comes back, "In homestead and in cottage they still dwell in England." They are straightforward, unpretentious, honest, hospitable people whose virtues are as much the backbone of England as the Pennines in which they live. I do not suppose many of them felt the need to leave the beautiful dale of the River Tees and that is perhaps why William Dent's letters were kept and carefully handed down. They provided a window on a world so full of danger and romance yet totally remote from the family farms of Low Green (where Dent was born) and High Green. I was shown the letters by Mr. Ron Grimwood of Scunthorpe (who married into the Dent Family) because he recognised that the events they chronicled would be of great interest to me. I believe their historical value is considerable. It is rare indeed to find a collection of letters amounting to an entire correspondence between one man and several members of his family. It is doubly so when their author not only gives a glimpse into the life of a medical student in the early nineteenth century and the boredom of garrison duties in peace time but who also was present on the Walcheren expedition, at the Battle of Vittoria, and the siege of San Sebastian. Because he reflects the views of junior officers, I found myself actually irritated that the 9th. Regt. of Foot missed the Battle of Waterloo through being posted to America.

Despite the derogatory reference to Queen Elizabeth the Queen Mother's ancestor, Lord Strathmore in the letter dated 29th. October, 1820, it was the account of the siege of San Sebastian which made me feel the existence of the letters should be made widely known amongst historians because to the best of my knowledge it is the only account of this bloody, and unexpectedly protracted, engagement outside official despatches. On the other hand, to my surprise, it was the dated details relating to the way Dent proposed to avoid service with the Militia which was of special interest to the late Prof. John Western, the acknowledged authority on the Militia in the eighteenth century.

The letters have three distinct phases; Dent's student days from Oct. 1808–May 1810, his service in the Peninsular Wars, Sept. 1810–Oct. 1815, and finally his peace time garrison duties in the West Indies, Feb. 1819–1824 when he was drowned on his way back to England on leave. They have been transcribed exactly as he wrote them with no attempt to introduce modern spelling, expression or punctuation. Occasionally a word or group of words has had to be omitted because the original letters were torn at these points or a much used fold in the paper made the text illegible.

In my opinion the correspondence presents the events and scenes in it with vivid clarity. But in their writing Dent's letters unwittingly show us, through his own life and that of his family, the age of transition through which England was passing. Even though he aspired only to become a surgeon, a far cry from the status of the physician at that time, it could not have been cheap by any standards to become a Member of the Royal College of Surgeons in the early nineteenth century. Yet the profits of yeoman farming, presumably unaffected by the developments of the "East Anglian Revolution", were sufficient not only to keep the family in Mickleton but also to send him to a London teaching hospital. Also when we read of the revolution, wrought by canal and road improvements, Dent reminds us how rooted people were in their own parish. In the letter dated 20th. April, 1819 he refers to an officer he has met as being "almost a countryman of mine" coming as he does from Piercebridge. This place is approximately 30 miles from Mickleton but the man, who by this date has travelled thousands of miles by land and sea, sees this brother officer, fellow Englishman, as basically a foreigner.

Finally, perhaps as it should be, the Dent letters bring home to us how fickle fate can be. Here was a man who had come through many campaigns unscathed either by injury or illness. His assurances of good health are almost monotonous in their regularity but the notorious West Indies posting finally caught up with him too. His last writings are more melancholy and permeated with home-sickness. Gone are the days of the carefree subaltern who was for a short life and a gay one. Now came the desire to marry and settle down. But it was not to be. The letter from the War Office of 9th. March, 1824 was sent in reply to correspondence from his sister-in-law inquiring why his ship was overdue. It had in fact foundered during a Caribbean hurricane and the Napoleonic Wars veteran was drowned. Had he lived it is more than possible the letters would not have seemed so important to the family and this record, so fascinating to us, might well have been destroyed.

Leonard W. Woodford.
Lincoln College of Technology.

ACKNOWLEDGEMENTS:

I would like to thank Miss Mary Dent, Mr Christopher Dent, Mrs. Mollie Dent and Mr. and Mrs. Ron Grimwood for their help. I would also like to thank the late Prof.J. Western, Major-Gen.A. MacLennan, Curator of the R.A.M.C. Regimental Museum and Mr Frank Atkinson of the North of England Open Air Museum for their help in interpreting some aspects of the letters. Also, my thanks to Mr Alex Morrison for the genealogical diagram.

London Sunday 30th October, 1808.

Dear Mother,

I received your letter by Mr. James Bayles on Wednesday last, and am glad to hear you are all well, he had a very indifferent passage up to Town. I am now very comfortably situated, and has got extremely good lodgings with other two young Men, I took a room when I left Mr. Bayles's at 7s. per week, but I only stoped in it for one week, for two young Men had taken two Rooms upstairs, and when they came I agreed to go with them, so we have two Rooms betwixt three of us and we pay eighteen shillings a Week, we have a sitting room and a bedroom with two Beds in it. The Person where we lodge would take us all three to Board and Lodging for a Guinea and a half a Week each, or five and twenty shillings per week and find our own Coals and Candles, for everything is extremely dear here, but we thought as being three of us we could live cheaper by only lodging in the house and find ourselves of everything we wanted; I am kept very busy, for there is no time to be lost while here, the two young Men who I am along with are very studious and we are writing out the lectures that we hear till twelve or one o'clock every night. We are likely to be brought into a great deal of Trouble about the Militia, for they are taking in all the Names and I am afraid I shall be put to some expence, it is not the local Militia but the regular Militia, I think the best way for me to do is to get into a Club, as there is a great Number of the Students of the Hospital who subscribe so much a piece to it, I shall be obliged to go to Mr. Whithorne in a day or two to get £15 for if I subscribe to the Club, I don't know as yet what I shall have to pay. I should not have wanted it yet, but on account of this Militia business I shall want other £15 about February; I think to myself sometimes that you will think I am very extravagant but I am confident that I am not, for I have paid upwards of £70 for the Lectures I attandance at the Hospital, I have also got a new suit of clothes of Mr. John Bayles and a pair of Boots, which have cost me £10 for Taylors and Shoemakers are very dear; they charge £1/4/- for making a Coat, I have also been obliged to get several books and a case of Pocket Instruments which cost me £5 all the Money that I brought from Mickleton is gone except three guineas. I wish you could send me three or four pairs of those white yarn stockings which I brought from Durham and a coloured neckcloth, and two or three of the Pocket Handkerchiefs, you can put them in the wooden Box that I used to send my dirty Close in, and if you can put a pot of Honey, Salted Butter or a piece of Cheese to fill it up with it will be very acceptable for everything is very dear and I did not know Housekeeping was till now, you can put a letter in the inside and that will save a shilling carriage, put good directions on and nail it down and lock it, I can open it with the key that belongs the Black Trunk and sent it then by the Waggon or the heavy Coach direct for me at

Mr. Smalls,
No. 4 St. Thomas's Tents,
Borough, London.

I am Dear Mother Your affectionate Son
Wm. Dent.

London December 5th 1808

Dear Mother,

It is now five Weeks ago since I wrote to you, and I expected to have heard from you before this time, I mentioned in my letter that you would be so kind as to send me three or four pairs of those white yarn stockings which I brought from Durham, and some Pocket Handkerchiefs, and a coloured neckcloth, for if I bought them here I don't know where I should get them hemmed, and to send them in the Box that my dirty close used to come home in, and to fill it up with anything that you had, to send it either by the Coach or the Waggon, perhaps you may have done so, and it may be miscarried or perhaps you may have not received my letter. I also mentioned that I was likely to be put about with the Militia, but however that is all quietly over now, for we left our lodgings and went to live in another part of the Town, and when the balloting was over came back again. I told you that I had got very good lodgings, along with two young Men who belonged the Hospitals, they are both of them very steady and studious, one of them attended last Season, and we derive a good deal of information from him, as he is very clever indeed, we are kept close at work both night and day, writing out the Lectures. We have a great deal of practice in the Hospitals, and accidents are continually brought in, we have an opportunity of seeing them all, as our lodgings are only a few Doors from Guy's Hospital. Mr. Withorne would probably tell my Uncle Harrison that I had got £15 of him, and I dare say that you will think I am very careless, and dont care what becomes of my money, but however I can tell you, that I am really as careful as I possibly can, I am very well aware that at this time you can but ill spare it me, I asure you when I came away, I had no idea, that I should put you to so much expence, but if I had this Season and another over, I hope I shall be able to do for myself, and make you some amends; everything is excessively dear, three of us pay 18 shillings a week for lodgings, and we find ourselves of everything we want, when on Average it costs us five and twenty shillings each a week. If you have not sent the Box, be sure to Nail it down fast and let it be entered in the way Bill, and then if it does not come safe to hand, I can recover the worth, I have nothing more to say, but that I am very well, never was so well in my life, and London agrees vastly much with me, I have not had the least Head Ache since I came up.

P.S. I had almost forgot to mention to you that I am attending Midwifery and that I have had one Labour. I managed all tolerably well, and the Woman is doing famously now, I expect to have another shortly, but the worst of it is, we have to give them 5 shillings and find them with medicines till they are quite well.

Direct for me at Mr. Smalls,
No. 4 St. Thomas's Tents,
Borough, LONDON.

I am dear Mother Your affectionate Son
Wm. Dent.

London Dec. 8th 1808.

Dear Mother,

I wrote to you on Monday saying that I had not received the Box, but however it arrived the day following after it had been nearly a Month on the Road, all safe and everything in it very acceptable. You will be kind enough to remember me to my Grandfather, and tell him I am very much obliged to him for his kindness. You desired me not to take any notice of John Fallowfield, and what you said of him I dare say is very true, he happened to come into John Bayles's while I was stopping there, to see his brother Thomas, but I suppose John Bayles and he is not on very good terms. I thought that he then looked a dissipated youth, I have not seen him since and I dare say shall not see him again, so you need not be afraid of my keeping Company with him. I have seen his brother William, who I think is a very nice young Man, and also Thomas is doing very well, he is in high spirits, and likes London very much. I suppose Jane Fallowfield told you about Jack, if she be at Mickleton, be so kind as to remember me to her, but perhaps she has forgot there ever was such a boy as myself. I must try to conclude for I am in a great haste.

I am dear Mother Yours etc.
Wm. Dent.

London February 17th, 1809

My Dear Mother,

I received your obliging letter about ten days ago, and are glad to hear you are all well, as thank God I am at this present time; I was very much shocked indeed to hear that young Mr. Bligh had finished his short career in this world, I had not heard of it before I received your letter, I told Mr. John Bayles but he had heard of it three weeks or a Month ago, I suppose that his Parents will by very much disturbed about him. I have made all necessary enquiries concerning Mr. Thornbury, and am sorry to say that your own account is but two time concerning his Death, he has been dead sometime, and I am told that there will not be a halfpenny for any of his Creditors, this indeed is but poor consolation for my Grandfather, for £200 is a very large sum to be lost, especially at this time when his own Grandson is going with so much in regard to Education; he has left a Widow but I do not know whether any Children or not, I saw him a short while after I came to London, and at that time he looked very ill and much emaciated, and I thought he would not continue long. Mr. Ashley Cooper the Surgeon and Lecturer at St. Thomas Hospital, has received a letter from Mr. Knight, the Inspector of Hospitals desiring all the Students that possibly can leave town, for to go to different districts to attend and dress the sick and wounded soldiers that have arrived from Spain, for the wounded are so numerous and the Assistant Surgeons so scarce, that the poor men are actually lost for want of Surgical Aid. Mr. Cooper hoped that every young Man that could go would, for he looked upon it both as humanity and as a duty to do so at such an emergency, he said that they would have that practice which it was impossible they could see at present in London, and as it would be only of a temporary nature, not exceeding a Month or six Weeks, he trusted that it would not interrupt out studies; the young Man that lodged with us is gone to Plymouth, and the other would have gone too but he is a dresser at Guys Hospital which has prevented him, there is near fifty gone from these two Hospitals; however, I am going to Colchester, I and other seven set out tomorrow morning, I beg your pardon for not asking your leave before I went, but as it is on such urgent business I hope you will be led to excuse me, and that my conduct will meet with the approbation of yourself and all my friends. I assure you that if thought I would not have been benefited by it, I never would have attempted such a thing, we have our expences found both there and back and seven pounds a month. I told you in my last that I had got £20 of Mr. Whithorne; when I came up to London, I wanted a Watch very much, indeed found it impossible to do without one Mr. John Bayles went with me to a friend of his and we got an extremely good stop watch, it was to be £8.8s. and since I have received the above £20 I have had to pay for it. I have also had to get a pair of Pantaloons, a Hat, a Pair of Shoes, a Neckcloth and some Pocket Handerchiefs, and as I am going to Colchester and am seem very near, I was obliged to get other £20 of Mr. Whithorne today, I have been costing up my accounts and find that I have had £155 since I came to London, and that above £100 of it has been paid for Lectures, Close, Watch, Boots, Books and passage in the Coach. I shall write to you as soon as I can after I get to Colchester, and let you know all particulars, remember me to all friends, while I am dear Mother,

Yours affectionate Son,
William Dent.

Colchester March 5th, 1809

Dear Mother,

I am afraid you will think me idle in not writing to you before this time, but I have been extremely busy and this is almost the first moment I have been able to command. I arrived in Colchester a fortnight ago, and was very much surprised to find such a number of Men sick as there is; there are only five Assistants now at this place, two having been sent to Meely Barracks where there is likewise a great number of Sick; each assistant is placed under a separate Surgeon, I am placed under a very nice Man of the name of Hill who is Surgeon to the first Battalion of the fourth Regiment which is come from Spain, and in that Regiment alone there is one hundred and ninety seven Men sick and wounded in the Hospital, and half of this number I have to take care of myself. I am very glad that I came here for besides attending the Sick and wounded, we have the privelidge of dissecting those who die, and in London we could not get a dead Body under three Guineas.

Six men belonging the fourth have died within these few days; the disease I think seems to be getting under but I cannot tell whether we will be wanted longer than a Month, if not I shall go back to London. I am in very good health, shall be glad to hear from you as soon as you can make it convenient; remember me to all my friends particularly to my Grandfather and Grandmother Langstaff who I hope as well as yourself are in very good health.

I am Dear Mother,
Your ever affectionate Son
William Dent

Direct for me thus
Mr. Willm. Dent,
Hospital Mate,
Colchester Barracks,
ESSEX.

Colchester Barracks April 3rd 1809

Dear Mother,

I received your letter on the 21st ulta I am sorry you should put yourself into any fears concerning me; you have heard very wrong reports about the disease that we have at this time in Colchester Barracks; it is not the Plague nor any such thing, it is merely a Typhus it was brought on from the soldiers being exposed to the Cold and being weakened from not having a sufficient quantity of nutritive food proportionable to the quantity of fatigue and exercise they had daily to under go, however it certainly is contagious, but as to its having extended to the inhabitants of the Town, is what I never heard of till I received your letter, six Weeks ago we had upwards of two hundred Men belonging to first Battalion of the fourth ill and now we have but forty and half of that number are convalescents, but there are several Regiments in this Garrison that are very sickly indeed, both Battalions of the fortythird and the seventy sixth have a great number ill and several have died, and they continue to take a good many into the Hospital every Day, but that is not the case now with the Regiment that I am with; I state things just as they are doing otherwise would be wrong. I might be attacked with this Fever though not in contact with the Contageous, and I may escape as I have hitherto done though in the midst of it, Medical Men you know are always exposed to dangers of this kind, and they are more seldom than any other people attacked with Fever; I never had my health better than what I have now, and I hope I shall continue so, the same I wish to yourself and all friends; how long I continue here is uncertain, I may only have to stop till the 28th of this Month, or all the Summer, just as the disease mends; I shall be glad to hear from you as soon as you can make it convenient, but they are dreadfull scrawls *what you have sent me lately.*

I am dear Mother,
Yours ever affectionate Son
William Dent.

PS. Remember me to Cousin Anth. Harrison, since I came to Colchester I intended to have wrote to him as I know he is particularly fond of any news concerning soldiers as soon as I can command a little time I shall certainly write to him, but as you may well conceive I have had tolerable sharp work of it. WD.

Colchester Barracks May 15th 1809

Dear Mother,

I have anxiously looked for a letter from you, this some time past, but I have been dissapointed, as soon as you receive this will thank you to write to me. I am very comfortable and extremely well used where I am now and intend to stop all the Summer if I can, for if I come home it will be as so much time lost, if on the contray I stop here I am improving. The Fever is nearly subsided now but a number of the Men are affected with Inflamation of the Lungs indeed where there are such a number of Men together (and there are several thousands in this Garrison) disease of some kind is sure to be raging. I have a very good Room to myself and got it neatly furnished for 5s per Week, the furniture consists of a Bed, a Chest of Drawers, a looking Glass, A Carpet, and a Wash hand Stand, a very small quantity you will think for the Money, but is difficult to procure them as every officer has to find the same. I have a Servant out of the Ranks to wait on me for 2s. per Week, I

Mess with the Officers of the Regt, Breakfast is 1s, Dinner 2s 6d., Supper 9d. I have had several things to buy (Sheets for they are not allowed with the Bed) Towels, a pair of Boots, Pantaloons Etc. I am very much in want of a Suit of Cloths, and Close now are serious articles, for I understand it will take more than a Months Pay to buy a suit; it was not my intention to have craved for anything of you while I was here but I am obliged to lay by 5 Guineas for it will take that Sum for a passage on the Coach when I come home, and I am feared to lay out any of the Money I have by me at present, for my Pay is not sufficient to keep me, and if I should seem short I have no friend here that I could apply to, if you will send me a Note in your next which you may do with great safety, by tearing it in two and sending each half in separate letters but dont send both letters on the same Day, this is the way two of the young Men have received money from home and it came very safe, Remember me to my friends while I am,

Dear Mother,
Yours affectionate Son,
William Dent.

Colchester Barracks Sept. 12th 1809

Dear Mother,

I have the pleasure to inform you that I arrived at Harwich on the 10th inst. from Flushing which place I left the day before, I wished to have wrote to you when I was at Tussoes in South Beveland, but all the Letters sent to the Post Office there were opened by the Adjt. General and that is the reason why you have not heard from me before. I am still attached to the 4th Regt. though we have only the Sick with us here, to the amount of three hundred and twenty. I have been remarkably healthy the whole time, which I am sorry to say has not been the case with a number of officers several have died and the Men were buried by dozens, such a sickness I dare say was never known to prevail in the Army before; the landing at Harwich was truly an awful sight, several of the Men died in the landing and on the Beach, and the in habitants would not let them lodgings to the Sick Officers, but if they had a few of the hard knocks the People of Flushing have got, they would be more humane to their Countrymen. I intend to stop here a few Weeks and as soon as the commence in London, to go there, I hope you will write to me and say how my Grandfather and all Friends are, while

I am Dear Mother,
Your ever affectionate Son,
William Dent.

London January 29th 1810

Dear Mother,

When I left Mickleton I promised to write as this day Week past, but my not having got everything settled to my wishes, I was induced to defer it till now. You of course would hear what places we got in the Coach, and our journey was better than could be expected, although the cold was very severe, we got into London by 5 o'Clock on Tuesday Morning, I accordingly posted off to Mr. Whithornes with Anthy, and myself to John Bayles's, who I am glad to say are all well and were happy to see me; they were very sorry to hear of my Aunt Higginson's unfortunate case, and John B. could wish her to come to Town as the place for relief, but I am afraid it is too late for any good to be done, I should be glad to hear when you write how she is. My Uncle Harrisons People would be rather surprised when they heard that Anth. and I did not lodge together, but Anthy's office being situated in Holbourn, which is at least three miles from St. Thomas's Hospital, it became necessary for our own convenience that we should be nearer our separate place of Studies; Anthy has got very good and genteel Lodgings in Fleet Street at a Guinea per Week; I have also got good lodgings near the Hospital with another very pleasant young Man, we pay each ½ Guinea per Week and find everything else ourselves; Anthy and I frequently meet together at Dinner, We have seen Thos. Gibson, John Atkinson, Geo. Langstaff and several more acquaintances, who were glad to hear News from the North. I have drawn £20 of Mr. Whithorne, which of course you would expect to hear of, and the manner in which it is spent viz: A course of Dissections £5.5s., A Body £3.3s., A Dissecting Case of Instruments £2. A Hat £1.8s. I have also ordered a Suit of Cloths, and a pair of Boots and Shoes, which I shall not be able to pay till next time I visit Mr. Whithorne, I shall be glad to hear from you and remember me to all Friends while, I am

Dr. Mother,
Your affectionate Son,
Wm. Dent.

London March 5th 1810

Dear Mother,

Having a little leasure time on my hands just now I think it my duty to address a few lines to you. My Uncle Harrison I dare say will have heard from Mr. Whithorne that I have got £20 more of him, indeed you never hear from me but when I have been (needing/Accounting for) money I have paid eight guineas for a Suit of Clothes, and have been three guineas more out for Books and a Dissecting Gown. I have also got two pairs of Boots and two pairs of Shoes, and have also a great Coat making, these I shall be able to clear off the next time I visit Mr. Whithorne; it is not the living in London itself that is so expensive, but it is Cloths, and other necessaries of that description, for I am live well and comfortable, Lodgings, Victuals, Coals, Candles, Washing and everything included for two guineas per week. You may expect the box with the old clothes shortly. I shall send them off next week by the Waggon, there are a couple of hats, three waistcoasts, Breeches and Pantaloons and other articles. I have no news to inform you of for London is very still just now. I am glad to hear my Aunt Higginson is better. Anthn. Harrison is very well and we often see each other at Dinner, he desires as well as myself to be remembered to my Grandfather and Grandmother.

I am Dear Mother,
Your every affectionate Son
William Dent.

P.S. I shall not forget to send my father his Hats, and I think I can't do better than send him a Steel Pipe.

London April 12th 1810

Dear Mother,

I dare say you will be anxiously looking out for a letter from me, particularly as I had not sent the Box, and the disturbances we have had in London, might create some uneasiness in your mind, however I am glad to say all is tranquil now, though for four days it was a very alarming aspect, the number of Horse and Infantry Soldiers, constantly parading the Street, had the appearance of London being a captured City some few lives have been lost, and some wounded have been brought to St. Thomas's Hospital. By some unaccountable delay I have not been able to send the box till this day, however I hope it will arrive safe; and the Glass, Pipe, and Boot Jack, will meet my Fathers satisfaction. I khould like to have sent Kitt a gun, but I could not spare the money at this time. I got twenty pounds of Mr. Whithorne on Saturday last, and paid for my Boots and Great Coat, and am now clear of everything; I got a pair of pantaloons and a Waistcoat last week and I have left but £9 out of the £60 I have had since I come to Town. I called on Anthn. Harrison at his office yesterday but he was not in the (   ) he is very well; I wish you would write to me soon, and let me know how you all are and what you are doing; for I have not had a Post Letter since I come to town.

I am Dear Mother,
Your affectionate Son,
William Dent.

London April 22nd 1810

Dear Mother,

When I wrote to you last, I was under the hope of not troubling you again for some time, but finding that the Lectures in the course of six weeks, will be brought to near a finish, and thinking myself equal to the task of being examined before the Royal College of Surgeons, I have been induced to write these few lines to you; you will probably recollect my mentioning this circumstance to you when I was last at Mickleton; but at the same time I wish you not to mention it to anyone except my own friends, for if I should be rejected, it will be a disgrace upon me, and a strong symptom of my negligence and inattention; but on the other hand if I should pass my examination it will be the best mark of Industry. You must be aware that this will be attended with a good deal of expence, if I pass I shall have £22 to pay for my Diploma for what you call taking out my Degrees and other expences attending it, likewise if I stop six weeks longer in London I shall want at least £15 more to live upon, so that I shall want altogether £40. I am afraid someone will grumble at all this expence but I cannot help it, for it is actually necessary, I wish my Grandfather would allow £100 of what he intends me to go on this account, for I know very well you cannot afford it; my examination will take place on Friday Week, before which time I request you to write to me, as I shall not receive the money before I have your consent; Cousin Harrison joins me in respects to you, Grd. father and Grdmother and all friends, while I remain,

Dear Mother,
Your ever affectionate son,
William Dent.

London May 7th 1810

My Dr. Mother,

I have the pleasure to inform you of my good fortune in passing my examination on Friday night last, it has relieved me of a good deal of anxiety I assure you; and you may now congratulate yourself on having a Son *a* Member *of the* Royal College *of* Surgeons, *which is more than most of the Medical Practitioners in the North can boast of. I know very well you are anxious to hear of my settling somewhere, and I wish I could gratify you in this respect, but it does not accord with my ideas at all at present; supposing I should come home what is there for me to do, even if I should begin practice on my own account it would be several years before I could expect any established business; another thing my appearance is so much against me, for I am too young. I have got the £40 of Mr. Whithorne, My Diploma cost £22 7s. 6d, the remainder will be sufficient for my subsistance while in Town.*

I am Dr. Mother,
Your affectionate Son,
William Dent.

P.S. Give my warmest respect to Gr.father and all friends.

London May 21st 1810

Dear Mother,

My Cousin Bayles informed me the other day of the Death of Aunt Higginson it was what I had been led to expect from the nature of the disease; I suppose my Uncle Robt. will be very disconsolate, being now left alone, I also heard of the departure of Miss Monkhouse, it is sorrowful news, but we must all fall sooner or later in the same manner. On Friday last I passed my Medical Examination at the Medical Board office, and have again entered the Army, and I leave Town for Portsmouth this week, this will be nothing new to you, for by my last letter you would perceive I intended going into the Army again. I was obliged to get £10 of Mr. Whithorne today, for I am in want of Clothes and I could not go to a strange place with nothing in my Pocket, I hope you have received the Box I sent, Remember me to all friends.

I am Dear Mother,
Your affectionate Son,
William Dent.

P.S. I shall write to you from Portsmouth.

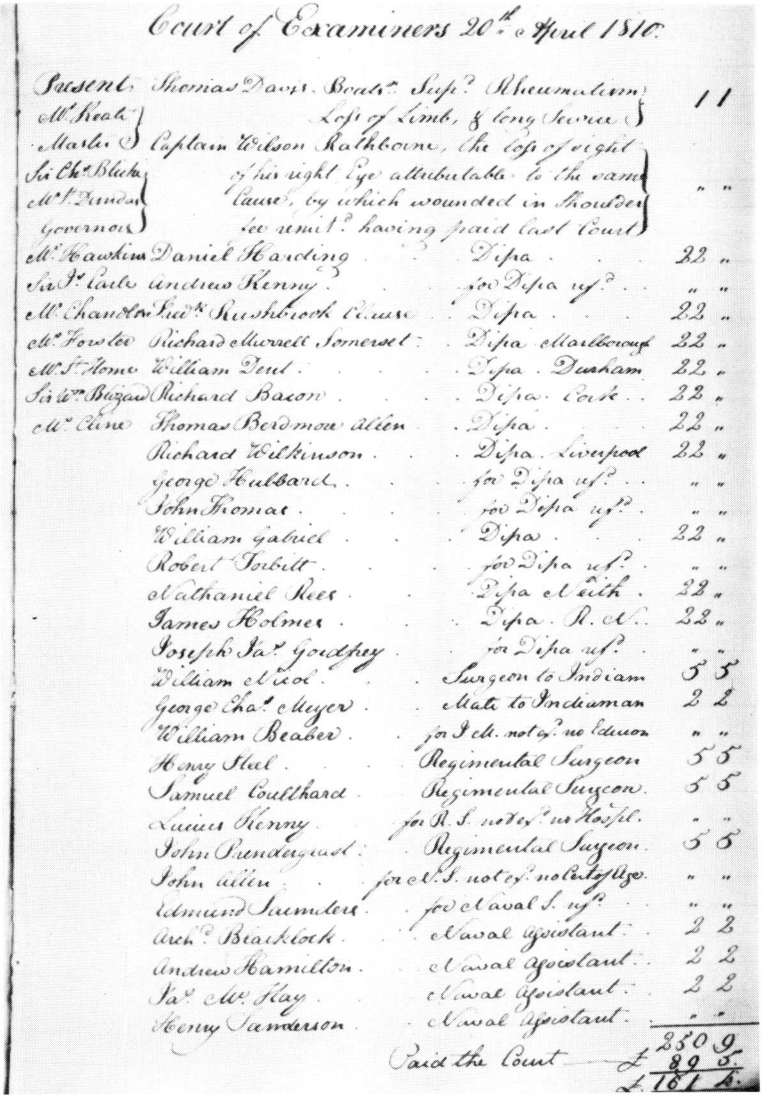

Court of Examiners 20th April 1810

Present			
Mr Keate, Master; Sir Chs Blicke; Mr Lt Dundas; Governors	Thomas Davis. Boatsn. Supd. Rheumatism, Loss of Limb, & long Service		1 1
	Captain Wilson Rathbone, the loss of sight of his right Eye attributable to the same Cause, by which wounded in Shoulder, fee remitd. having paid last Court		" "
Mr Hawkins	Daniel Harding	Dipa	22 "
Sir Js Earle	Andrew Kenny	for Dipa ref.	" "
Mr Chandler	Fredk Rushbrook Clarke	Dipa	22 "
Mr Forster	Richard Murrell Somerset	Dipa Marlborough	22 "
Mr Ev. Home	William Dent	Dipa Durham	22 "
Sir Wm Blizard	Richard Bacon	Dipa Cork	22 "
Mr Cline	Thomas Berdmore Allen	Dipa	22 "
	Richard Wilkinson	Dipa Liverpool	22 "
	George Hubbard	for Dipa ref.	" "
	John Thomas	for Dipa ref.	" "
	William Gabriel	Dipa	22 "
	Robert Torbitt	for Dipa ref.	" "
	Nathaniel Rees	Dipa Neath	22 "
	James Holmes	Dipa R.N.	22 "
	Joseph Jas. Godfrey	for Dipa ref.	" "
	William Nicol	Surgeon to Indiaman	5 5
	George Chas. Meyer	Mate to Indiaman	2 2
	William Beaber	for I.M. not ex. no Educn	" "
	Henry Steel	Regimental Surgeon	5 5
	Samuel Coulthard	Regimental Surgeon	5 5
	Lucius Kenny	for R.S. not ex. no Hospl.	" "
	John Prendergast	Regimental Surgeon	5 5
	John Allen	for N.S. not ex. no Certe of Age	" "
	Edmund Saunders	for Naval S. ref.	" "
	Archd. Blacklock	Naval Assistant	2 2
	Andrew Hamilton	Naval Assistant	2 2
	Jas. McKay	Naval Assistant	2 2
	Henry Sanderson	Naval Assistant	" "
			250 9
		Paid the Court £	89 5
		£	161 4

Page from Court of Examiners Book at the Royal College of Surgeons

Hilsea Barracks Near Portsmouth
June 24th 1810

My Dear Mother,

I intended to have wrote to you soon after I come here, but by delaying a short time longer, I thought would put me in possession of something more to say, but unfortunately that is not the case for I have little news to communicate. I have been here near a month, there are very few sick, not more than Eighty in Hospital, and nearly ten Medical Men to attend them which makes the duty very easy and comfortable, much more so than when at Colchester Barracks. I hope you don't fret at my entering the Army. I am perfectly happy, and I see no reason why you should not be so, for I think the Army an excellent School for a young man, who has a desire to excell either in his Profession or to become acquainted with the manners of the World. I am recommended to the Medical Board for an Assistant Surgery by Dr. McGregor, but whether it will succeed or no I cannot say, if it does I shall take care to let you know. I suppose by this time you have begun with Haymaking, and if you have no better Crops than we have here, I am certain that none of you will be killed either with Raking *or* Forking *The weather has been remarkably hot, and scarce half an hours rain for this month past. The Durham Militia are come here from Portsmouth, they expect to march shortly for their own County. I have seen John Stapler once or twice, but I believe he is now gone into the Country to work. I think I have scrawled over what little news I know, and I must try to conclude with my best respects to my Gr.father and Gr.mother and all our own family, in the mean time believe me to be*

Dear Mother,
Your ever affectionate Son,
William Dent.

P.S. We have had a very particular operation today. Taking the arm off at the Shoulder Joint.

Portsmouth July 1st Sunday Morning

Dear Father,

I have just time to inform you that I am ordered to Gibraltar with the 82nd Regt. and the Signal is now flying for all hands to be on Board, otherwise I should have given you more information on the Subject.

I beg to remain with Love to all friends,
I am Dr. Father,
Your ever affectionate Son,
William Dent.

Gibraltar September 17th 1810

My Dear Mother,

A Packet being about to sail for England, I have the pleasure of addressing for the first time since my arrival at this place, which was about five weeks ago, after a long but a tolerably pleasant passage. I wrote to my Cousin Harrison and desired him to inform you of my arrival; The Packets not being very regular I had not a possibility of writing till now, but you may assure yourself that I will not be negligent in this point, you shall hear from me every Month or two. Gibraltar is a strange place, and strikes the Spectator at first sight with a degree of astonishment not easily to be conceived; it was very hot here at first coming, but is now like the Summer in England. I have had my Health extremely well, and the Headache has troubled me but once, which I was afraid in a warmer Climate would occur oftener; I am in want of nothing, I am supplied with the Clothes, and Money I have plenty, my Pay is Nine Shillings per Day and my expenses not more than five, I hope this will make you and all my friends as easy in your Minds as I am, for I assure you I want nothing; Fruit in particular is cheap here, Grapes, Peaches and Figs at 2d per pound. I saw my Name in the Gazette of the 4th August as Assistant Surgeon to the 9th Rgt which is stationed here, but I have had no notification of it yet from the Medical Board, very probably I shall by the next packet. News is very barren here although the theatre of War is not very far from us, and we are obliged to the English Newspapers for every information; About a Week ago a Regiment of French Deserters were landed here from Carthangena, they are upwards of a 1,000 strong, all fine young Men, and have as fine appearance as any Rgt in the British Service, I hope you will write to me soon, I must try to conclude with my Gratitude to my Father, Grd Parents and Brothers while

I am Dear Mother
Your ever affectionate Son
William Dent.

Gibraltar November 27th 1810

My Dear Father,

A Convoy being about to sail for England I avail myself of the Opportunity in writing to you, which I should have done before if the Packets from this place had been more regular; I expected to have heard from Mickleton or from my Cousin Harrison by the last Mail but was disappointed; I have not had a letter from England since I left it myself (except one from the Medical Board) which makes me feel anxious to hear from you. I am now appointed Assistant Surgeon in the 9th Rgt Foot, a very fine and deserving Corps, the Appointment took place on the 2nd August last. You probably have seen accounts in the Newspapers which might alarm you, concerning the Plague having made its appearance in this garrison; however you may be easy on that Subject, for I believe Gibraltar was never more healthy than it is at this time; there certainly was a Fever of a Contageous Nature broke out in some parts of the Town, and likewise in the 7th Veteran Battalion, but proper measures were immediately taken, and the People who were attacked with the Disease, were encamped on the Neutral Ground, on the Spanish side of the Garrison however since then we have had no communication with Spain and all vessels arriving from the Spanish or Portugese Coasts, are put under strict Quarrantine. I wrote to my Brother about two Months ago and likewise to Aunt Harrison, but having received no answer, I am afraid they have either been lost or detained. I am sorry to say since that I have been employed on a very unfortunate Expedition, one in which I don't believe that British Soldiers behaved with so much determined Cowardice. The Army (if I may call it as such) consisted of 300 Men of the 89th Rgt with 60 Artillery Men and 4 Pieces of Cannon, about 500 Germans, deserters from the French Army and a Spanish Rgt we took in at Ceuta, making in all upwards of 1,500 Men, and commanded by Lord Blaney, with this force we were to attack Sebastian and take Malaga; we landed on the Morning of the 14th October 20 Miles from Malaga, and about 10 Miles from a Castle which was in possession of the French, and it was thought necessary to be taken before we advanced any further; with this intent a Flag of Truce was sent which the Commandant of the Castle answered by firing on it. The force we had (except the Spanish Regiment,) was immediately brought within Musket Shot, and commenced firing, which was kept up till after dark, when the firing ceased; we had 3 or 4 Men killed and some wounded; Major Grant was shot in the Neck and died afterwards; during the Night the Cannon had been landed and by daylight were ready to play on the Castle, but with little effect; about 12 o'clock, Lord Blaney, perceiving he could make little or no impression on the Place, was going to take up another position, when a Column of French Infantry Cavalry made their appearance, which being joined by the People in the Castle, immediately attacked us, drove the Artillery from their Guns and took them, the whole retreating in Confusion for ½ a Mile, when the 89th rallied drove the French back and retook the Guns; the French being dressed exactly like the Spaniards, cried out (Hispaniola) signifying they were Spaniards, which induced Lord Blaney to go up to speak to them, when they instantly laid hold of him fired a volley among the English and put the whole Army to the run; then commenced such a scene of Confusion as I never witnessed, some endeavouring to get into the Boats, others even attempting to swim to the Ships, and if the Rodney Man of War had not brought her broad side to bear on the Beach, and commenced a heavy fire of Grape, most part of us would inevitably have been taken. We have no late arrivals from Lisbon but I believe both Armies continue in the same position, I think there is little doubt but Lord Wellington will ultimately be driven out of the Country. I have nothing further to communicate but that I am in very good health and perhaps more comfortable than I should have been as Assistant to any Surgeon near home; I shall be very happy to hear from you, but in the meantime remember me to my Mother Grandparents and Brothers who although I am far from home receive the best wishes of

Your ever affectionate Son
William Dent

Gibraltar March 17th 1811

My Dear Father,

By the last Packet I received your Letter of the 4th Jany. and am excessively happy to hear that all friends at home are doing well, it has relieved me from a good deal of uneasiness, for I had some Idea that you never intended to write to me again. I am happy to hear my Cousin Harrison is expected to commence his Profession at Barnard Castle shortly, I thought he would not have neglected writing to me till now; if he is returned into the Country remember me to him, tell him, he has my best wishes, and I hope his success will exceed all your expectations, for I entertain a very high opinion of his Abilities. I am very much delighted with the Idea of your improving the Lundhill, but I believe it will tend to your own interest as well as mine; tell my Grandfather Dent, that I think it would make a more compact thing of it, if he were to dash a few more acres to it, then who knows but I may spend my Cottage Days *there, though it is in a* bleak *situation. I can perceive by my Mother's letter, that she is still in the same fretting way, tell her that her notions about being bound for life are all frivolous; I have a regular Commission (which by the by cost me 5£) from his Majesty, which I am at liberty to resign when I think it convenient; I live very comfortable, and with respect to Close and Money, I am much better off than when I left England. Before this reaches you, you will have heard of the Action which took place between Cadiz and Chiclana; it was as honourable to the English as it was disgraceful to the Spaniards who behaved shamefully; they were not even brought into action, but remained in a Wood till the business was over; Two Companies of the 9th were there, they had four Officers wounded and nearly half of the Men. A Body of French from the direction of Malaga, made their appearance in front of this Garrison the other Day, but after exacting contributions and burning a few houses they retired. You must excuse this bad writing for I am a good deal hurried, I beg leave to remain with respects to all friends*

Dr Father
Your ever affectionate Son
Willm. Dent.

Gibraltar August 21st 1811

My Dear Father,

I have been expecting to have heard from you for some time past, but have been vexatiously disappointed, very likely you have wrote to me, but Letters frequently miscarry; however a Mail for England closes to Morrow morning, which induces me to give some little account of myself, since I last had the pleasure of writing to you. I believe I wrote to you on the 17th March last, giving you some trifling account of the Action at Banosa, next day, three Assistant Surgeons and myself belonging to this Garrison, received orders to embark in the Papillon Sloop of War, and proceed to Cadiz, to attend wounded French Prisoners, on our arrival there, we found these unfortunate Creatures, in a most wretched condition; I think without exception the ugliest Wounds I ever saw, numbers of them having fractured Limbs from Grape Shot, and not being dressed for three days after the action (on account of our own wounded being so numerous) they really had a frightful appearance, and to crown all, they were laying on the floor, it being impossible to procure Hospital Bedsteads in sufficient numbers. The Duty was very severe for about a Month, but having an apportunity of seeing such practice and performing operations, was an equivalent to all hardships of this kind. I remained in Cadiz till the 15th June, when I received an order to hold myself in readiness to return to Gibraltar and join my Regiment, which I was very sorry for, as Cadiz of all the Places I ever was in, is the most charming. About this time a small expedition was fitted out for the relief of Tarragona which offered me an opportunity of returning to my Regiment where I hoped to have a little rest (but variety is the Life of the Army) and I had not been an hour in Gibraltar, when our Regiment received an order to embark next day and accompany the expedition; we accordingly embarked and sailed for Tarragona on the 21st June, after a fine passage of six days we arrived at our destination, but to our Mortification found the French had carried every out work, and made their approaches within Pistol Shot of the Town. Communications having taken place between the English and Spanish Commanders the latter declined any assistance, saying it was impossible to keep the place three days, if the French opened their Breaching Batteries, which they did that Evening, and played incessantly the whole Night and next day; about five o'clock in the Evening, one of the English Men of War Telegraphed that the French Lines were manned, and presently after that they were advancing to the Breach; The Spaniards now commenced firing from the Walls and Tops of the houses, but the French having mounted the Breach, drove them out of the opposite end of the Town in less than half an hour, when to the number of several thousands, they made their way down to the beach with the hope of being taken off by the Boats, but none being there, they went along the Shore, perhaps thinking to get through some part of the Enemy's line, and escape into the Country, but the French who foresee everything sent down their Riflemen and opened two Field Pieces on them which completely brought them to a halt, their Cavalry then charged and hewed down the Spaniards on all sides, taking the whole Prisoners, it was now so dark we could observe nothing from the Ships, but the French set fire to the Town which burnt for several Days after. The Town being taken we had no further business, but for three or four days after we sailed up and down the Coast, making demonstrations of landing, mainly with the intent of harrassing the enemy we then made the best of our way to Port Mahon in Minorca, to Water and Provision, we remained there a Week after seeing the Antiquities of the Island we sailed, and arrived in Gibraltar the 26th of July. We have little or no News; but accounts have reached us that a Contagious Disease is raging at Carthagena, in consequence of which all communication with Spain will be cut off to Morrow and every Ship from the Mediterranean put under Quarantine. Will thank you to write to me on the Receipt of this. I beg leave to be remembered with particular affection to my Mother, Brothers and all friends, while

I am Dear Father
Your ever dutiful Son
William Dent

P.S. Will thank you to enquire of Any. Harrison if the Box I left in London is still there or was sent to Portsmouth when I left England; if in London let it remain there.

Gibraltar May 21st 1812

My Dear Harrison,

I had long ago given up all Idea of ever hearing from you, but by some good fortune or other I yesterday went into the Military Secretary's Office, and found a Letter from you, dated even as late as October, 1810; though it is so old, you cannot imagine the satisfaction I felt, at seeing the hand writing of my old Companion and Relative it infused me with new Spirits, and I could have wept for joy. I had a letter from my father in Feby. last, saying you had wrote several times to me, but none have come to hand, the one mentioned above excepted; it is useless writing home for I have nothing to communicate which can be interesting to them, further than, that I am perfectly well, and desire to be remembered to all, which you will have the goodness to express. I never knew this place so excessively dull as it is at present, not a syllable of News. The Troops which formed the Garrison of Tarifa from

Gibraltar, have all been withdrawn, and replaced by Detachments from Cadiz under Coln. Gough; this arrangement has taken place in consequence of the impropriety of Genl. Campbells ordering Coln. Skerrett to defend the Town to the last, for the Town is only surrounded by something like a Park Wall; I have reason to be sorry for it, as for the last two Months I have been Acting Surgeon there and received extra pay. Ballesteros is in Cantonements about three Leagues from this, his Cavalry had a trifling affair with Soults the other Day, he took five prisoners and sent them into Algesiras with the Epulets of the Commanding Officer. I think the Affairs of Spain wear a more favourable Aspect than they did three Years ago, and if the Spands., persevere, there is not the least doubt but they will ultimately succeed in expelling the French beyond the Pyrenees. The middle and lower Class of Spaniards are worthy of everything that is great, and if their Armies were well Officered, they would make the French repent ever having entered the Country. Desertions from the French Armies continues very great, I have seen them come into Tarifa by six and seven's, in general they are very fine Men, well dressed, and their appointments peculiarly good; I am sure I don't exaggerate, when I say there has been brought to this Rock within the last two Years, not less than seven thousand Deserters. We are in great expectation of having Lord Wellington down towards Seville and Cadiz, it would be the Salvation of Spain if he could raise the siege of the latter place.

I regularly examine the Marriages in the Newspapers and am astonished I don't perceive your Name, but I should hope, ere, this, you are made a Happy *Man for Life. It gives me great pleasure to hear you are continuing your Profession under such favourable circumstances, you have every prospect of becoming Independent in the course of a few Years,—as for your humble Servant a short Life and a pleasant one.*

Do of all things, write to me, and let me know a little North Country News—you all seem to be little short of Republicans.

Believe me to be Dear Harrison
Your ever sincere friend & Cousin
William Dent

Gibraltar September 8th 1812

My Dear Cousin,

I should have answered your letter of the 15th June long before this if I had not been impressed with the Idea of the Regiment leaving this place for Portugal, and we have been under orders for Field Service nearly three Months, and still are so, but the report now is, that we cannot go until relieved by some weak Battalion from Lisbon, however when we do embark, I shall let you know, but I am afraid we shall Winter in Gibr. I was extremely sorry to hear of the destruction of the Mill, it certainly is a severe loss, but I hope it was insured to nearly its value. With respect to the long details of Deaths it is truly Melancholy, it is sufficient to depress the Spirits of any Man who is not possessed of an unusual strong set of Nerves, if I should return home I imagine there is not a Schoolfellow left to recognize me. I have not wrote to my Mother for some time, the fact is, when I attempt it, I never can make out more than three or four lines, and Gibraltar News must be very insipid to her, you will be kind enough to inform her that I am perfectly well and not in want of anything (which by the by) is no small consolation, since I have made no demands for two Years and a half past. This Diabolical Rock is once more shut out from all intercourse with the World, in consequence of some vague reports of fever, and all arrivals are put under quarantine. You have long ago heard of the defeat of Marmont the effects of which are now operating on every corner of Spain, Soult has broke up from before Cadiz, drawn in his Detachments from Malaga, Ronda, and the Country around here, he is concentrating the whole of his force, which it is imagined will be near forty thousand Men, has proclaimed to the Spaniards that he is marching to chastize the English General, and will then return and protect them from all insult; I hope he will share the fate of his Brother Marshal, however that a Battle will take place in a very few days is inevitable. Genl. Cruz and Col Skerrett entered Seville the other Day, and took two or three hundred Prisoners, as to Ballesteros we don't hear a word about him; The Expedition from Minorca I believe still remains at Alicant without attempting any thing, it is nothing near so strong as was at first represented, Genl.

Whittingham who has the organization of our Army at Majorca informed the British Government that he had 8000 effective Men, but when Genl. Maitland received them he could produce little more than 3000. The (   ) there is a great deal of knavery carried (   ) amongst these kind of people.

I cannot conclude without wishing you every happiness which the Married State *will* admit *of, and at the same time beg you will present my best respects to your Lady.*

I am Dear Cousin
Your sincere friend
William Dent.

Gibraltar Novr 27th 1812

My Dear Mother,

I have sit down three or four different times within the last Month, with a determination of writing to you, and as many times something or other has disappointed me, however a Packet leaves this for England to Morrow and I cannot let slip the opportunity of sending you this scrawl and informing you that I am both in good Health and Circumstances. I have not had a Letter from home for a considerable time, which convinces me there is great irregularity in the Post Office, for some of you must have wrote within the last six Months. My last Letter from Any. Harrison is of 15th June, but everything in it, wore such a dismal countenance, (his own Marriage excepted) that it was nothing more than a series of Deaths and Misfortunes; I should be glad to know how he goes on though I intend writing to him by the first Mail after this. My reason for delaying writing so long, was, that the Regiment being under orders for Portugal, I thought it would be the wisest plan to send you a line or two when we were actually embarked, but however that order being now done away, I cannot form any excuse for my negligence; two hundred Men are drafted from this

Battalion to the first, and letters from Col. Molle, who is on leave of absence in England mention the probability of another detachment being shortly sent, when the remaining part of this Battalion will be ordered to England to recruit, this I dare say you will happy to see prove true, but for my own part I can live much better in Gibraltar than in England. Letters from the Army received a few Days ago mention our first Battalion to have lost six or seven Officers and upwards of an hundred Men killed and wounded, composing part of the Rear Guard in the retreat from Burgos, this gives strength to the report of our sending more Men to them. News from this place you need not expect, for we are as much separated from all the World, as if we were encamped on Mickleton West Pasture; the only thing of a political Nature worth mentioning is of Genl. Ballesteros who has refused to serve under Lord Wellington, he is consequently deprived of the command of his Army and sent to Ceuta a place considered as a receptacle only for the worst of Criminals, he wrote several letters to the Regency at Cadiz, couched in very mutinous language. I am glad to find the Walcheren Prize Money is likely to be paid, my share will be about 12£. which is no trifle these hard times. I hope the Plot of Ground at Lund Hill is gradually improving, I assure you I often think of it, and if I live as long, intend to spend my Cottage Days there; Brother Kitt *it is expected, pays every attention to it, but from his great partiality for* Rabbits *and* Ducks, *I have my doubts of the fact. I am excessively sorry to hear of the death of my Grandmother, and I am afraid my Grandfather has felt the loss severely, remember me most kindly to him, for I owe every thing to his goodness. With respect to myself, Dear Mother, you must not be under any apprehension, I have every thing which can make me comfortable in regard to Clothes and Money and believe me I live with a body of Officers who are perfect Gentlemen. I beg leave to conclude with my most sincere regard and well wishes to all friends and relatives.*

While
I am Dear Mother
Your affectionate Son
William Dent

Villa Real, near Lamego, 17th Feby. 1813

My dear Mother,

My last letter to you was dated from Lisbon, which I hope you have received, and wherein I mentioned the probability of my soon joining the Army, and I now have the pleasure of informing you that we left Lisbon on the 20th January, went in Boats up the Tagus about seven Miles, and after twenty six Days of pleasant marching, we arrived at this place, about three Miles from Lamego; the weather has been very fine, and the Roads good, a very fortunate circumstance in our favour at this season of the Year. Lord Wellington has joined the Army, but there is no symptom of its being collected for some time yet, in consequence of the number of sick. Since I left England, it has always been my constant hope that I would never more be a drawback on the Affairs of my family, but however, Necessity has no Law, and I am obliged to request you will let me have 20£, the way I can receive it is as follows, my Uncle Harrison must write to Mr. Withorne in London, to deposit that Sum in the hands of Mr. James Window, Agent for Army Hospitals, No. 5 Craigs Court, Charing Cross, who I know and can draw on him for that Sum, you will very probably ask what I can want with Money here, the reason is, that it is impossible for me to be either like the other Officers of the Regt. or actually to do my duty unless I have two Animals, one for Baggage the other to ride, which I am not able to buy at this time without some assistance; you will be kind enough to inform me as soon as possible, if you can conveniently comply with my request, remember me to all my friends, who I hope are in as good health as myself, Believe me to be

Dear Mother
Your affectionate Son
Willm. Dent.

If you have not received my former letter,
direct for me with
1st Battn. 9th Regt.
5th Division
Lord Wellingtons Army
Portugal

Camp, near Villa Neuva,
4th June. 1813

My Dr. Cousin,

I have been guilty of a breach of friendship in not writing to you long ago, but as nothing particular as yet has occurred in the Army that perhaps may plead in my favour; and as it is uncertain when another Mail leaves this I shall keep this letter open and give you a Journal of our operations. We broke up from our Cantonments on the 14th May, and six divisions passed the Douro at different points, we continued our march through the Traslos Montes, the worst Roads I ever saw, our Artillery suffered much; the Towns we passed through were Villa Real, Mourca, Mirandela, Outeiro, Alcanizes, Carvajalas, where these six divisions closed in and Lord Wellington joined us, we were happy to find that our Cavalry had taken 250 of the French Rear Guard at Salamanca. On the evening of the 27th ult. Genl. Picton was ordered to pass the Esla with the third and fifth Divisions, however it was not fordable at the point we went to, and were obliged to return to our ground we previously occupied, the Cavalry crossed lower down, but several Men and Horses were drowned; a Squadron of the enemy's Cavalry remained behind to reconoitre our numbers, they were immediately pursued by our Hussars and the whole were run down in less than a league; on the Morning of the 28th a Pontoon bridge was thrown over the River, and the divisions passed in succession, we continued our march, leaving Zamora and Toro on our right; and we are now within five leagues of Valladolid; on the 2nd. inst. the 10th Hussars had a brilliant affair, took the whole of the 16th French Cavalry Regt. with very little loss, they mistook the English for Portugese but paid dearly for their mistake, the Colonel of the 16th was killed. The Army at present is in admirable condition it does not consist of less than seventy thousand Infantry, the Cavalry are likewise very strong; the Hussars have made them quite jealous of one another. Genl. Graham with the 1st and 5th Divisions forms the left, Genl. Picton with the 3rd and 6th. forms the Centre, Genl. Cole with the 4th and 7th forms the right, the whole under the Eye of his Lordship; and if I may be allowed to hazard a speculation, we will be on the Ebro in three Weeks. June 5th. We entered Rioseco, this morning, it is a very large old town, the enemy left it at three oClock yesterday Morning, consisting of ten thousand infantry and a thousand Cavalry, they have gone in the direction for Palencia, which is eight leagues from this; they give out, that they dont intend facing us till once across the Ebro. Genl. Hill has marched on Avila, and cut off the communication between the Armies of the North and South. This is all the News I can recollect at present, tho their are various reports of our Cavalry having taken more prisoners. A Spanish Army I understand is a few leagues on our left, but as yet, we have seen none of these worthy Dons. *Since we entered Spain the Weather has been very sultry, but the Country is one continued plain, and of course very few Men knock up from the march, I can add nothing more as the Man is waiting for the letters, remember me to all friends, and be assured I will write to you whenever anything particular occurs. Tell my Mother I am in very good health and Spirits,*

Believe me to be
My dear Cousin
Your sincere friend
Wm. Dent.

Camp in front of Salvatierra
25th June. 1813

My Dear Cousin,

I wrote to you last from Rio Teco and since that time have had but one days halt, which has prevented me from writing to you earlier; The whole of the Army arrived at Palencia on the forenoon of the 7th, the French rearguard under Genl. Boyer, had but just left it; Joseph Buonaparte, received the troops there the day before, he remained three hours, and retired in the evening with the whole of his infantry on Torquemada, the high road for Burgos, in the neighbourhood of which some skirmishing took place, always to our advantage. We crossed the Carrion on the 8th and on the 10th the Pisuerga, halted on the 12th. at Sotiesgurdo, more on account of provisions than anything else, for the troops have been on half Rations for several days; On the 13th the French dismantled Burgos, to the great joy of those who expected to make up their last account in front of it, but as we from the left Column, have not had the pleasure of seeing it; the whole Army moved by the left and our Column crossed the Ebro, on the afternoon of the 14th. at Puente de San Martin, it would have been impossible almost to have crossed, if an enemy had been before us, but he had not been aware of our passing at that point, and had taken up position near Pancorbo, I believe the whole Army was across the River on the 15th and continued its march on Medina, where it was again collected; nothing took place till the 18th when the enemy about five thousand strong, took up a position near the village of Osma, the Ground was well chosen, and he had a small River in his front, however he was driven from it in a very short time by the 1st Brigade of the 5th. Division, and Horse Artillery, we suffered some loss in killed and wounded, the enemy retired on the high road for Vittoria, we continued our march on the 19th. and 20th. on the Morning of the 21st. the baggage was ordered to remain in the Rear, and it was said the French intended to meet us at Vittoria which proved correct; however it would be nonsense my attempting to give any account of the battle, when you will see every thing much clearer by the dispatches, for Officers of Regts. know very little about an action except what is going on in their own immediate front; the French had an immense Artillery which they played with great effect; on this day he also had a small river in front, which was only fordable at some places, on the right of his line he took possession of a village and a bridge over the River, posted about fifteen thousand Men in rear of it, with Cannon on both flanks, it was evident, that if he was pushed at this point, he must lose everything; the 5th division was ordered to storm the town, and foolishly went down in close Column of Regts. instead of in line, the consequence was that every Cannon Shot told, and the division lost a great number of Men, however they took the village most gallantly, and soon afterwards the bridge, and the enemy retreated at all points, pursued by our Cavalry until dark, we have taken One hundred and fifty pieces of Cannon, several Millions of Dollars, besides Silver and Gold Bars, the whole of Joseph Buonapartes and the Baggage of the french Army; what prisoners are taken I dont know. I went into Vittoria on the Morning of the

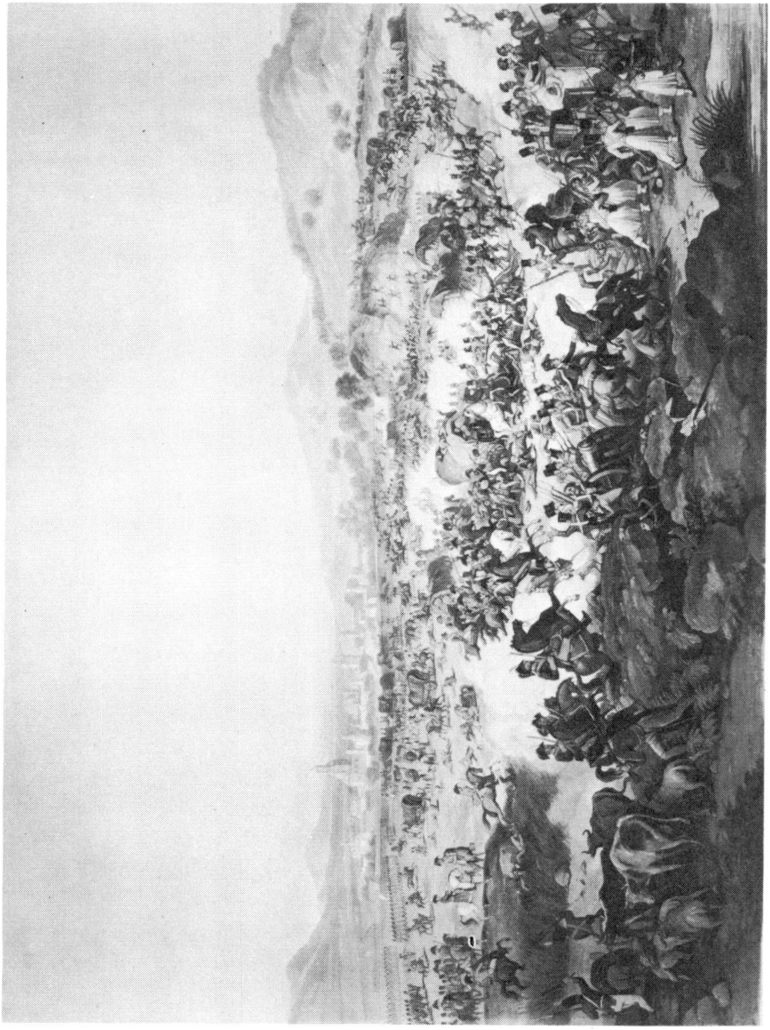

'The Victory of Vittoria' by I.M. Wright

22nd and unless I had actually seen it, I could not have believed that such destruction could have taken place, hundreds of fine french Carriages, Cannon, Ammunition, Waggons, Carts and Mules, were laying in the Roads, Ditches and Fields for Miles round the Town; I have seen several private Soldiers, with Bags full of Dollars selling them for five to a Guinea, their not being able to carry the Dollars. 26th June Genl. Graham with the 1st Division went in pursuit of Foy's Corps, which had retired on the Bayonne Road pressed him very hard, and took his only Gun; the other part of the Army under Joseph retired on Pamplona, left a garrison of five thousand Men, and has gone in the direction of Roncesvales in the Pyrenees, Genl. Hill's Corps I am told is to break ground before Pamplona, but there are so many stories *going, it is dangerous believing anything we dont see. 27th Our division countermarched to Salvatierra and on the 28th arrived at Penna Ceurada, joined the 6th division, under Genl. Clinton; we are encamped near the main Road from Vittoria to Logrono, to watch Marshall Suchet, and Genl. Clausel, who have a considerable force there, 29th. The two divisions, (5th and 6th) marched for La Guardia, when within a league of that place, an order came for the 5th division to again countermarch and support Genl. Graham, who is at Tolosa; 30th. Arrived at Vittoria, went over the ground on which the action was fought and counted 180 pieces of Cannon taken the whole are not yet brought in. It is said that Clausel is hemmed in at Tudela, and cannot escape, whether this is true or not I cannot say, but several divisions are in that direction after him; 1st July. Marched to Mondragon, on the road for Bayonne, the French have left a garrison of 1500 Men in San Sebastian, which I should think would be easily taken. 2nd July. We halt this day at Mondragon, we have been marched till we scarce have a leg to stand on; there is not a word of News stirring in the Camp this Morning, we march in the Morning for Villa Real de Alava. I have not had a letter from you or from any of my friends for a long time, nor have we any late News at all from England, I am afraid Matters are not so prosperous in the North of Europe, as they were some Months back.*

You must remember me kindly to all my friends, particularly to my Mother, I know she will construe everything about into the worst light, but I am perfectly content with my situation. I shall write to you by every opportunity

Believe me to be
Your sincere friend and Cousin
Wm. Dent.

San Sebastian 9th Sept. 1813

My Dear Cousin,

Two Months have now elapsed, since I wrote to you last, which was from Mondragon and I have received no letter from you, I can only attribute this to the uncertainty of the Mails, for I have not the least doubt, but you have wrote to me oftener than once during that period, however I hope I shall hear from you soon. Some short while ago I received a letter from your Sister, at least it was wrote by her, but I rather think it was not altogether her composition, upbraiding me for saying, I would never more write home, and I should certainly have answered it before now, if it had been more settled times with us, but since we came before this place, we have been constantly stunned with the roar of Cannon, and as you are always anxious to hear of Military Matters, I shall give you a short account of our misfortunes and also our successes *before St. Sebastian: Our division relieved a Spanish division before it in the early part of July, and broke ground before a fortified Convent and redoubt, outside of the Town, a Battery of six Eighteen pounders and two Howitzers, played against it for three days, but the Frenchmen would not stir from it, a Portugese Brigade was ordered down, for the purpose of what Military People call Feeling the Enemy but they met with so warm a reception, they were obliged to retire with loss: the next day the same brigade was ordered to storm these outworks, supported by the 9th Regt. the enemy were driven from the Convent and Redoubt, though considerable reinforcements came to their succour from the Town, and our Regt. distinguished itself; we were now enabled to break ground before the body of the place, but it is necessary you should have some idea of the situation of the place, which is the strongest*

Fortification I ever saw Gibraltar excepted; it is nearly surrounded by the Sea, on the Sea side is an immense high mountain, with a strong Castle on the top, at the bottom of this Mount is situated the Town, both sides of which are washed by inlets of the Sea, the front of the Town, consequently is very narrow, and amazingly strong, it consists of two lines of defence and a regular Glacis; the outworks being taken, the trenches were carried close up to the Town, and the Wall was breached at the angle next the inlet, which could only be got at, at low water; on the Morning of the 24th July, the troops were in the Trenches by three oClock ready to storm, but the enemy had made so large a fire inside the breach, it was thought impossible to enter, and they accordingly returned to their Camp; they were in the trenches by four oClock on the Morning of the 25th and the signal being given, they moved on towards the breach, but from some fatality or other, the troops that advanced first were not well supported, and they were cut to pieces, the remainder retired into the trenches, and the business finished by a furious Cannonade; our loss was from four to five hundred killed and wounded; the next morning the enemy made a successful sortie and took some prisoners: There is one thing I am sorry to see in the English Newspapers about a Lieut. Coln. Campbell, who is said to have behaved gallantly, whereas there is no such Man here, and the praise bestowed on him is intended for a Lieut. Colin Campbell of our Regt. who led the forlorn hope and was wounded in the breach; this unfortunate assault took place at the very time of the fights between Roncesvalles and Pamplona, when orders were received to embark the Artillery forthwith, this put all of us in consternation, but the glorious issue of the aforesaid Battles, again revived our drooping spirits, and it was determined, the siege should be prosecuted with redoubled vigour; in the meantime I left the division, and embarked at Passajes with wounded Men for Bilboa, and arrived there after an uncomfortable voyage of ten days; Bilboa is the finest Town I have seen in Spain with the exception of Cadiz, I left it on the 16th August, and arrived before St. Sebastian on the 21st where everything was in the greatest forwardness for enlarging the former breach, on the 26th the Batteries opened and on the 31st the breach was reported practible, at 12 oClock in the

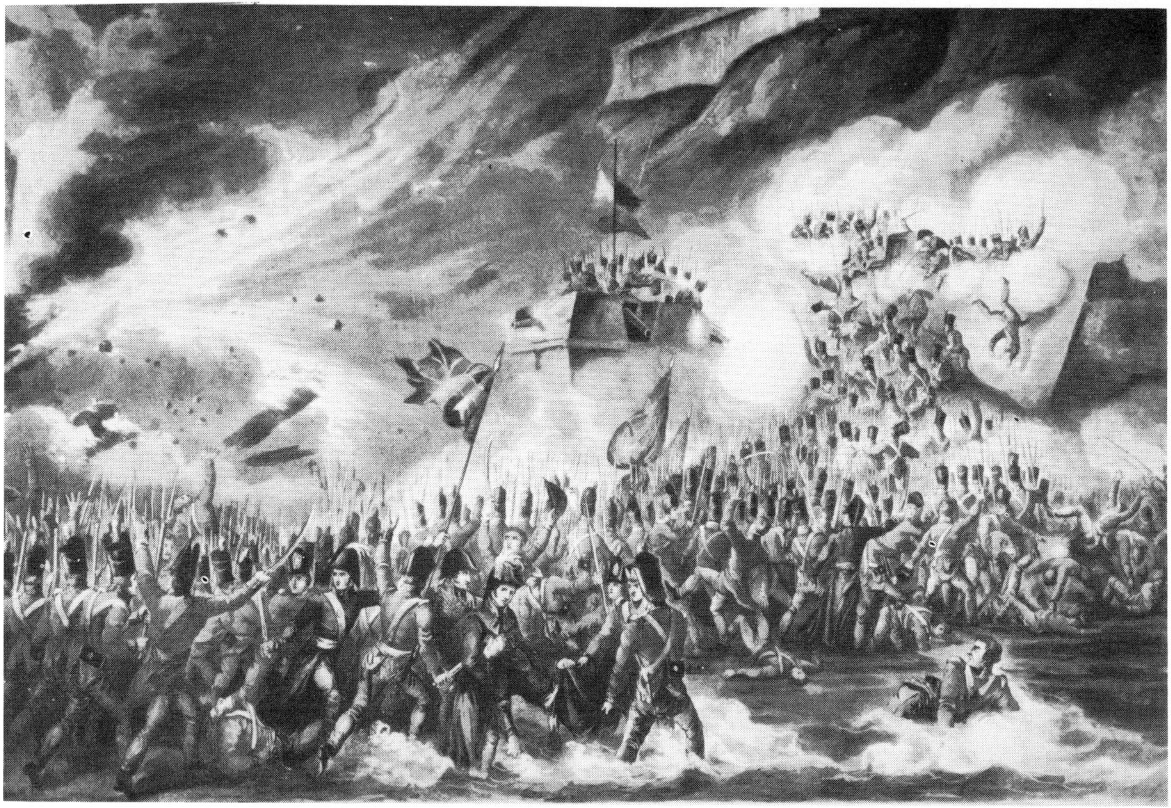

'The storming of St. Sebastian, August 31st., 1813'

day the attack was made, and for nearly two hours the most obstinate fighting took place in the breach, at length the enemy gave way, and he was driven from Street to Street into the Castle, all the Streets were barricaded with Barrells filled with Sand, and Room left for only one Man to pass at a time so you may imagine under what disadvantage the English fought; it was a most horrible sight I was looking on the whole of the time till the breach was forced; I believe we have lost about 1500 Men and many valuable Officers, the enemy maintained himself in the Castle till the evening of the 7th; on that Morning sixty two pieces of Cannon opened on it, and would soon have beat it to the ground; the Governor therefore surrendered himself and Garrison prisoners of War, Officers to retain their Portmanteaus and Soldiers their Knapsacks, and to be embarked at Passajes for England when Transport can be provided, so after two Months, fatigue and hardships we are now quite Masters of St. Sebastian.

Tell my Mother I hope she is well and not uneasy on my account, for I never had my health better, give my best respects to those who enquire after me, and particularly to your Sister and Mrs. Harrison, and

Believe me to be
Your most sincere friend and Cousin
William Dent.

Camp before St. Jean de Luz
22nd October 1813

My dear Cousin,

I don't know whether I ought to upbraid you for negligence, or attribute it to mischance, my not having received any letter from you for such a length of time; but that no neglect may be laid to my charge, I write you this, and hope that it may have a safer passage than any you may have wrote lately, merely for the sake of informing my friends that I am well, and also to convey a little Military News to yourself. I wrote to you last from St. Sebastian which place we left on the 24th Sept. and marched to Oyuzun, where we remained until the 7th Oct. it had been reported a few days before that we were to make an invasion into France and on that morning the divisions were under Arms at two oClock, we cautiously moved towards the Bidasoa, a River which at this part divides France from Spain, our division was to cross between Irun and Fuenterrabia; along the course of the River are a number of Dykes to prevent inundation, behind which the troops were hid until low water; the enemy must have been completely deceived for he had no force near the River, except his Picquets, who immediately on the English fording, fired their Muskets and other signals of alarm and fell back on the Main body in the Rear; the River in some places was very deep, and numbers of the Men lost their Firelocks, and others narrowly escaped being drowned, but however once across the enemy was driven from position to position as fast as he could take them up, and only in one instance made a stand; our Regt. being more in advance than any other of the divisions immediately charged, and they gave way; we had ten officers wounded and near Seventy Rank and File killed and wounded, (without vanity our Regt. behaved well that day): The enemy were pursued about two leagues, when orders were received to fall back, and the position we are in at present was taken up; the left resting on the Sea, and extending along a range of Hills across the Bayonne Road into the Pyrenees as far as the Eye can reach; the heights have been crowned with Redoubts, and our position is altogether very strong; it has been a matter of surprize to many why we have remained so long inactive, the enemy is making himself much stronger every day in our front; they are working incessantly and I am afraid it will cost us a good number of men to force their present lines. The two armies are not more than two miles distant, the outposts close together, but don't molest each other. The inhabitants have all fled, and I don't think I have seen a real frenchman in the Country. The Weather has been very bad, and a few days will determine whether we advance or retire, for it will be impossible to bear up against Wet and Cold; perhaps if Pamplona falls, which is expected in a few days, we may venture further into the Country, and look out for Cantonments, the Country appears level and as it is reported that our Right will be able to turn the enemy's left I hope our cavalry will do something decisive in the plain. I don't know when a Mail leaves this and will consequently have this open a few days.

25th. A Mail goes off this evening, but I have nothing new to add, we are still in the same state of inactivity. Remember me to my Mother and all my friends.

I am Dear Cousin
Your sincere friend
Willm. Dent

N.B. An English Mail was delivered yesterday but it brought nothing for me.

Cantonments, two leagues from Bayonne.
21st Novr. 1813

My Dear Mother,

I know you will think me idle in not writing to you long ago, but I have regularly corresponded with my Cousin Harrison, and was confident that you would hear of me and of all my proceedings, so that it was on that account, I did not write earlier; but not having received any letters from my cousin for several Months, I feel rather uneasy, and am at length induced to send you this scrawl. I received a very instructive kind of a letter from S.H. some time ago, unbraiding me very justly, for what I had said in my last letter to you, however what I said, was not intentional and I hope will be thought no more of. I can not make out the reason why none of your letters have come to me, as I cannot doubt you having wrote to me. We are at present about seven Miles from Bayonne, the whole Army is Cantooned in small villages, and Farm Houses in the Country, but whether we are to remain in them for the Winter, I know not; I think it very improbable while we have so active an emeny in front of us; they still have one division on this side of Bayonne, and the other day some sharp skirmishing took place with the Outposts in which Genl. Wilson and Genl. Vandeleur, were wounded. I shall not say anything of the attack on the French lines, on the 10th inst. our Column was very little engaged, the enemys position was turned, several miles to our right, and consequently know very little about it; the Dispatches are the best information. The inhabitants had fled in great numbers on our advancing; they had been given to understand by the French General, that those who remained behind would be murdered, however that not being the case, whole families are returning daily. The Discipline with regard to the protection of inhabitants and their property is much stricter, than ever it was in Spain or Portugal which very much displeases the Soldiery of those two Nations; St. Jean de Luz is a very neat town and a tolerable good market in it; Head Quarters are there at present. I wrote to you on the 13th but afterwards tore the letter, as positive orders were given that no Mail would be made up till this day. When you receive this I hope you will not omit writing to me as several interesting circumstances must have occurred, of which I am ignorant. I wonder why one of my hopeful Brothers is not able to say something, but I suppose they are so much employed in Farming, that the whole of their Ideas are consolidated in the pursuit of that Art only. I shall be happy to hear that all my Friends are well, to whom I beg to be kindly remembered, particularly to Mr. & Mrs. H. Jun.

I am dear Mother
Your affectionate Son
Will Dent

Bident. 11th March 1814

My dear Mother,

It would be useless my attempting to make any excuse for my Idleness in not writing to you, on the receipt of my Brother John's Letter, which I received about six weeks ago, therefore you will attribute my long silence to negligence alone, (this is a very hopefull confession from the Son to the Mother). I was exceptionly grieved to hear of my poor old Grandfathers death, but from his decay and Years in Life I had in some measure expected to hear of his decease by every letter from home, for the Epistles that are sent me, generally contain nothing else, but a series of Melancholy News. You particularly require to know how we live in this Country, and a great many other things which you ought to know nothing at all about, however to gratify you I will give you a recent History of them. If a Man has plenty of Money, he may live well, almost everywhere, but if he has not Money, then he is obliged to bite the hob, and live on a Soldier's Rations, which to be very concise with you is as follows (per Day). One Pound of Biscuit, One Pound of Meat. two Ounces of Rice and one third of a Pint of Spirit; but Officers generally live in Messes of three or four together, and with a subscription of four or five Pounds each a Month in addition to the aforesaid Rations, you would be surprized to see how comfortably every thing goes on. All fresh comers to this Country, unless they are Men of private fortune, are obliged to live on little more than their Rations for several Months, in consequence of their being invariably paid in advance, previous to their leaving England, and this Army at this moment is only paid up to the 24th August. 1813. Every kind of Wearing Apparel may be had at St. Jean de Luz, from English Sutlers, which follow the Army, and also Tea, Sugar, Butter, Hams, and everything the same as in England with the exception of paying a little dearer; I hope the account I have given you, which I assure you is perfectly correct, will dispel those Nervous Qualms, *to which I know you are habitually subject, and not imagine that I am starving in an enemy's Country.*

I have not heard from My Cousin Harrison for a long time, and I cannot account for it, unless he is busily employed in Rocking the Cradle, that he cannot find time to write; tell him that I perceive Marriage is a very dangerous undertaking, when it has made him forget the Companions of single life. However I shall write to him very shortly.

As to Military News, you will I dare say know more particulars about the Movements of this Army, than I do myself. Our Column under Sir John Hope, remain to beseige Bayonne, and six Divisions of the Army about the middle of last Month, moved along the course of the Adour, crossed it and have beaten the French in two or three battles, in the last of which it is said the French Army was completely dispersed, and has fled towards

Toulouse; Lord Wellington I believe is at or near Bourdeaux; in the meantime we are very quiet here, doing little or nothing. The 1st Division threw a Bridge across the Mouth of the Adour, with the assistance of the Navy, (a great many of which were drowned in the attempt) and have broke ground before St. Esperet; that Fort being taken, the Town will then surrender or be knocked to pieces; We have about ten thousand Spaniards with us under the command of Don Carlos de Espania, they are very fine looking Soldiers, and I hope will behave well.

We are amused every now and then with the talk of Peace, I should think this Summer will decide it one way or other, but I don't think Buonaparte will give in, as long as he has a friend to stand by him. I hope you will make some of those lazy people at home, write more frequent, and not such dry scraps as John sent me, but I suppose they are not much in the habit of letter writing; You will remember me to all friends at home and at Bd. Castle, and believe me to be

Dear Mother
Your ever affectionate Son
William Dent

Camp at St. Rhone near Bordeaux
June 2nd 1814

My Dear Cousin,

I received your letter of the 15th ult. a few days ago, and must confess, that the subject of it, is serious, and not to be disregarded; however I have weighed the matter well in my own Mind, and am very certain, that if I was settled in private practice, even superior to what I could expect, that at the expiration of one Week, I should wish to be in the situation I am in at present; I have a horrible dislike to be running fidgetting after a parcel of old Women. Since I wrote to you last (which is a long time since) I have spent a very pleasant life in the neighbourhood of Bayonne, and after the Gates were opened had an opportunity of seeing it, and also marching thro' it, when we received the order to move to this place, which was on the 15th of May; the Country is very level and nearly the whole way to Bordeaux is a continued forest of Pines, from which the Natives were hard at work extracting the Turpentine. On our arrival here, we were given to understand that an expedition was going to America under Genl. Hill, and Nineteen of the most effective Regts. in this Army were collected for this purpose, when orders were received from England for Ten Regts. only, to hold themselves in readiness for immediate embarkation, which were Brigaded as follows, 1st Brigade Genl. Kempt. 9th 37th 57th 81st. The 2nd Brigade Genl. Robinson 3rd. 5th. and 27th. the 3rd Brigade Genl. (   ) 4th. 44th. and 85th. the second and third brigades have already embarked, and we march tomorrow morning for embarkation also; where we are going, no one here has the least idea, the most prevalent report is that we rendez-vous at Cork, but you know more about it than we do.

Bordeaux is a charming town, and living very cheap, we are laying in Sea Stock for six weeks. When at Biarritz I had a letter from my Mother, you will oblige me by telling her of my receiving it, and of the obligation I feel myself under from her kind offers, but that I am not in want of any assistance at present, also that I have drawn the Money from Mr. Window some time since.

If we go on any interesting expedition I shall write to you, but I think this manouvering is only to frighten the Yankees.

With best respects to all friends,
Believe me to be
Your sincere friend
Will Dent.

P.S. When you write, you never mention whether you have got a Son and Heir yet or no.

Kingston, Upper Canada. 10th Octo. 1814

My dear Mother,

The last time you heard of me I believe would be from my Cousin Harrison, to whom I wrote previous to my embarking at Bourdeaux, which place we left on the 16th June, on our voyage for North America; after a pleasant voyage of seven weeks we arrived at Quebec on the 8th of August, but were not permitted to land in consequence of the wind being fair, to take us higher up the river; we landed on the 10th of Augt. about thirty miles above Quebec, and commenced our March for Montreal, where we arrived on the 21st Augt. The weather was very fine, and the accomodations on the road very good, and the beautiful appearance of the Country on both sides of the River, led us to hope that we had not made a bad exchange between Europe & America. Montreal is a very large and pleasant Town, but everything exceedingly dear; we left if on the 1st Sept. for Kingston; and a very uncomfortable march we had of it. It is supposed we remain here for the winter, which I hope will be the case, as the Country above Kingston has been much destroyed by the Americans. The whole of the Army now regret very much our ever having left France, the people are very uneasy and everywhere imposition is attempted to be practised on us. You must have heard before this of the Affair on Lake Champlain, and the retreat of the Army before a handful of Americans which caused about five hundred English soldiers to desert; everything is carried on in a very different manner to what we had been used to in Europe, and every one is discontented.

The Fleet at this place is nearly fit for Sea, one of the ships carries 102 Guns, the other four are smaller; they have taken in Stores and Provisions for the Army on the Niagara frontier, and I suppose will attempt to elude the Americans, and deliver their Cargo before they risk an action, as the safety of the Army and the Country above Kingston depends on the success of the first combat. Genl. Prevost is expected here every hour; what his object in coming to Kingston is, I don't know, perhaps he wishes to make an attack on Sackett's Harbour, if he does I hope the success will be different to that of Plattsburgh.

I am afraid it will be a longtime before I hear from you, letters are two or three Months in coming from England, but don't neglect writing on the receipt of this as I am anxious to know how everything goes on, at home, for I often think of Mickleton & B. Castle though I am four or five thousand Miles off I am in very good health, and I have been ever since I came to the Country, though in the Autumn, Ague is very prevalent here, but the frosty weather has commenced which will soon dispel the cause. Remember me to all friends, who may enquire after

Your ever affectionate Son
William Dent.

You must direct for me in
Upper Canada
North America

Portsmouth. 4th Augt. 1815

My Dr. Mother,

I have the happiness of addressing you from this place on my arrival from America; we arrived here the day before yesterday, I should have wrote to you immediately but we were uncertain as to our landing, and this Morning's Mail has brought us the Order to proceed direct to Ostend, we shall sail as soon as the Wind is favourable. My Dr. Mother I hope this intelligence will not add to the inquietude, which I know you have constantly entertained for me as for my own part, I should gladly have shared in the glorious Campaign of the Army we are going to reinforce but from the existing circumstances I should think the affairs of the Continent will soon be settled. Perhaps you might have thought me negligent while in America in not writing to you oftener, but the Postage in that Country is exceedingly slow, and I had nothing particular to mention except my (Health) which has invariably been good. Now that I am nearer home you shall hear more frequently from me. I am very anxious to hear from you, but do not write till you hear from me again, when I shall be able to direct you how to address me; with best wishes to all the family & Relatives

I am Dr. Mother
Your affectionate Son
Wm Dent.

Ghent 13th Augt. 1815

My Dear Mother,

We sailed from Portsmouth on the 5th and arrived at Ostend on the 6th. we were immediately landed, and after marching two or three Miles, again embarked in Boats which brought us to this place by the Canal from Bruges, nothing can exceed the kindness with which we are treated, nor can I express the pleasure I feel in being removed from that miserable Country America, to one where we can enjoy every kind of luxury. This Town is very large and contains a great many curiosities worthy of attention particularly the paintings and Sculptures in the Cathedral. On Friday next (the 18th) we commence our march for Paris, going by the route of Mons, Cambray, & Bavay, but at the same time there is a report that the troops lately arrived from England are not to quit Belgium, which I hope is not true, as every one must have a wish to see the French Capital.

I hope you will write to me, on the receipt of this, and give me all the News you can collect, I wish very much to know how my Cousin Harrison is getting on, we have both been very remiss in not corresponding with each other. Remember me affectionately to my Father and Brothers, and any other, who may take the trouble to enquire after your ever affectionate Son

Wm. Dent.

PS. You must direct for me as before with the Duke of Wellington's Army
France.

St. Amand 4th Dec. 1815

My dear Mother,

I have delayed writing to you till now, in consequence of my not having made up my mind as to applying for leave to come to England, but as the season is so far advanced, I think it will be the most prudent plan to defer it till the beginning of April. The Regiment returned to this place on the 24th of October, and all of us are exceedingly comfortable again, and I think it probable we shall not be moved before next Summers encampment. I hope you have been more fortunate in your harvest than the miserable wretches in this Country for I never saw such an unfavourable season as it has been, and the distress it has made all around us is very melancholy. I am very much obliged to the person you mentioned in your last letter, for the favourable representation he made to you in my favour, I only hope he was right in his judgement. You must excuse my writing so short an epistle, as nothing has occurred worth mentioning, and my only object is to let you know I am in good Health, and expect to be with you in a few Months.

Remember me to all the family, and believe me to be

Your ever affectionate Son,

Willm. Dent.

Ecoueir near Paris, 17th Dec. 1815

My Dear Mother,

When I wrote to you last, the Army was in Camp, it broke up on the last day of October, and was cantoned in the Villages arround Paris, our Regiment occupied the Village of Boulogne, about three Miles from Paris, where we were very pleasant and comfortably quartered. Everything has been very quiet, and nothing of consequence taken place except the trial of Marshal Ney, whose sentence was carried into execution on the 7th inst. According to the treaty of Peace, all the British Troops that were to leave France, have marched for Calais and Boulogne and the remaining thirty thousand have been reformed into three Divisions, each Division consisting of three Brigades; our Regiment remains in France and still in the third Division, so that when you write, you will direct to me as usual. This miss formation of the Army caused the whole of the cantonements to be changed, and we left Boulogne on Monday last, for this place which is about ten Miles from Paris; it is said that we are not to remain here long, but to occupy the fortified Towns on the frontier, mentioned in the Treaty.

As you are the only person in England, with whom I have any correspondence, I must fill this letter, with enquiries after those who probably have forgot me; with respect to my Cousin Harrison, your last letter gave me great satisfaction, on hearing of his deserved success in his profession, as also the happiness I know he must enjoy in his domestic life, for I was not aware that he had become a Father, till I received your letter; you will give my kind respects to him and all his family, as also my Uncle and Aunt Harrison; I hope most sincerely your predictions will not prove correct about Sally and do not fail to let me know how she is in your next. If I recollect right you mentioned that Mr. Kitt was on the look out for a Wife, this piece of news, certainly astonished me amazingly, but it is now near six Years since I saw him and must naturally suppose he has left off all idea of sucking the Pap*; had it been John my surprize would have been much less, for he was always famed for an amourous disposition. How do my two Uncle's at the top of the Hill make it out, I dare say much the same as when I left Mickleton, their mode of life does not admit of much variation. When you write let me know if the Farm's are in a progressive state of improvement, and particularly the one at Lund Hill.*

I do not recollect any thing more I have to say or enquire after, but that my Finances are tolerably good, my Wardrobe very passable and my health never better, remember me to my Father, and any one that may enquire after.

Your ever affectionate Son
Will Dent.

Camp at Ene near Valenciennes
18th August 1816

My dear Mother,

When I wrote to you last, we were at St. Amand, in the hope of remaining there quietly for the Summer, but as this Army is liable to be called upon to act in the field at anytime it is necessary that we should be a little unused to Camp, consequently we are all under Canvas, we should have been so long ago, had not the extraordinary wet weather prevented it; I find you have had in England also a very wet season; When I found that we were actually going into Camp, I applied for leave of absence to England for three Months, thinking to avoid it, but the answer was that no leave of absence could be granted to a Medical Officer, till after the Camp had broke up for Winter Quarters, which I suppose will be about the middle of October, and as yet I have not made up my mind, whether I shall make a second application then or not; if I do I shall ask for four Months. Your last letter astonished me a little about Uncle T's marriage; some People as they become older certainly do not become wiser. I perceive by the Newspapers that Cooks Bank at Sunderland has stopt Payment, I hope you are as fortunate in this instance as in the one you mentioned in a former letter. How are our friends at Barnard Castle passing their time, I should like to have a glance at them, without being seen, I hope no misunderstanding has arisen amongst you, by you having desired me to direct my letters to George Barkers. Do you know whether John Bayles lives in the same house in the Strand as when I left London. I left a Trunk with him which I wish to call for if I should come to England (by the bye) some time ago I perceived his friend Headlam's name in the Column of Bankrupts, this I am afraid was not from unforseen misfortunes but from making a more splendid appearance in the World, than his resources could afford.

When you write to me, pray let me know all the little Country News; some things which you think little or nothing of at home perhaps may be very entertaining to me here. Remember me to all our family, and any other that may enquire after

Your ever affectionate Son
William Dent.

To George Dalkin Bombr.
Capton F. Gordons Camp
3 Battn. Rl. Artillery 1 Division
British Army Cambry

Daymes near Cambray
12th Dec 1817

My dear Brother,

It is now some time since I received your letter and I intended to have answered it earlier, but something or other has always prevented me from so doing. I was not surprized at the melancholy account of my Uncle James's decease, I thought from his appearance the last time I saw him that he would not have lived so long as it appears he did; I think my Aunt was perfectly right in coming to Mickleton, as the society in which she will be, may in some measure allieviate her affliction, you must let me know how my brother John and Bessy are doing, and if there is any appearance of an offspring; at the same time remember me kindly to them. When you see Anthy Harrison and his Wife, give my best respects to them, and also the Children; for although he may appear to have acted negligently towards himself, and ungratefully to his friends at home, yet I shall always feel the greatest friendship for his attention to me while at Barnard Castle. I am also anxious to know if Matrons affair is drawing to a crisis; and if Billy the brother was ever got shot of. I must not forget to mention about the Mare, she answers tolerably well as a Roadster but I have been several times out hunting with her in which she was so violent, as to be in a white lather all the day, but as we are now prevented from hunting in consequence of the young corn I intend getting her into good condition in the Spring and parting with her. Do not forget when you write to let me know about the Oliver's and if (   ) left them, and also how Dixon is going on. With respect to ourselves we are not so comfortable as when we were quartered at St. Amand, the Regiment occupies ten different Villages, and they are so dirty that it is impossible to go outside of the door without being up to the knees in the Mud; everything appears quiet, and it is said we shall return to England next Year, which I hope is not true.

Remember me to all friends up the Hill especially to my Uncle Wm. and also affectionately to my Father & Mother,

Believe me to
Your ever affectionate Brother,
Willm. Dent.

Direct for me as undermarked
Mr. Wm. Dent,
Assist. Surgeon,
9th Regt. of Foot
France.

Camp Cambrai
18th October 1818

My Dear Mother,

I have refrained writing to you until this present time in the hope of being able to inform you, whether we should quit this Country or not, and as it is now decided upon, I shall give you an idea of our proceedings, & probable arrival in England. We shall march from here on the 21st to the neighbourhood of Valenciennes, near which place we shall be reviewed on the 23rd by the Sovereign; we shall return to this place on the 24th and remain one day; on the 26th we shall commence the march for Calais, but I do not expect to be in England before the 8th or 10th of November, as much delay must necessarily take place in the embarkation of so large a body of Men, but immediately on our arrival I shall write to you and inform you of the place we are likely to be quartered at, which we have every reason to believe will be Canterbury. We have been encamped here since the 2nd June and have had the finest Summer ever collected; the only fault, it was a little too warm. You had better not write to me until you hear from me again.

Remember me to all the family and friends.

Believe me to be
Dear Mother
Your affectionate Son
Willm. Dent.

Gosport 2nd Feby. 1819

My dear Brother,

As we shall embark tomorrow Morning, I have a few leisure moments to write to you previous to my leaving England; in the first place I must acknowledge the receipt of your letter, and to express my grief at the sudden and unexpected dissolution of my Brother John's partner; it was an event so unlooked for that I was almost thunderstruck at reading it, and I am certain must have produced the greatest affliction to you all; I was also much alarmed about my Mother, but as you mention that her health had somewhat improved, I trust that your next letter will confirm its perfect reestablishment; you will of course give my most affectionate love to her and my father; to whom I shall write after we are settled in the West Indies; at present we are ignorant what Island we shall go to, but you may depend on hearing from me. Everything here is in a bustle, I have been occupied all day in getting Baggage on board; the 4th and 54th regts embarked yesterday, and sailed this Morning with a fine Wind, and if it should hold in the same quarter we shall sail on Thursday.

I thought I had mentioned to you about the Mare in a previous letter, she did not turn out so well as I could have wished although I sold her for more that what she cost me, I afterwards bought another and when I embarked at Calais I only got Seven Pounds for him; I have sold the Grey Hounds for Eight Guineas. You will excuse my not writing to you a longer letter; but my next will I hope be more lengthy and interesting.

Remember me to all friends and believe me to be your

Affectionate Brother,
William Dent.

St. Vincents, 20th April, 1819

My dear Mother,

When I wrote to you last from Gosport, we were on the point of embarkation; however contrary Winds prevented us leaving Spithead until the 28th of February, we had a very favourable breeze and made the Island of Madeira in eight days and arrived at Barbados on the 3rd April without experiencing even a gale of Wind; I have always been particularly fortunate in my voyages by Sea; but in this instance nothing could be more pleasant. We remained at Barbados six days, were landed and received by Lord Combermere, G.C.B.; half of the Regiment is quartered here, and the other half is divided between Dominica and St. Lucia, these two latter Islands have the character of being unhealthy, but St.

Vincents I believe is one of the best Islands in the West Indies it appears to me something like Gibraltar as to climate, but we have always a breeze of Wind which prevents the heat from being oppressive, the Barracks are situated about a Mile from the Town of Kingston but as the Road to it is very steep, and we are not yet being supplied with Horses, we have had little communication with any of the Planters who have the character of being uncommonly Hospitable. The appearance of this Island is very romantic, the interior is mountainous, and covered with Woods to the very summits; the Valleys and Lands along the shore are all cultivated with Sugar Cane by swarms of miserable looking Negroes. I am under great obligations to my brother Kitt for his last letter and I hope he will continue to give me every information as to Country News; for the further a person is from home, the interest becomes greater, even in trifling events; I want very much to know how Watsons business has terminated, and if poor (   ) was done out of his money. I forgot in my last letter to mention that we have lately got an Officer into the Regt who is almost a Countryman of mine, his name is Mills, his father lives at Piercebridge he knows all the Country round, and we have frequent conversations about Durham & Yorkshire he is also perfectly acquainted with the West Indies having been here before, they have a very fine Estate in St. Kitts; he has got two months leave of Absence to go and see it.

I shall write to you about once in two Months, as this is not a place from which you can expect much News, my only object is to let you know how I am. You will remember me to all friends at Barnd. Castle and at Mickleton; they are so numerous I cannot particularize.

I remain my Dear Mother,
Your ever affectionate Son.
William Dent.

Address as under:
Assistant Surgeon Dent,
9th Regt. of Foot,
St. Vincents,
West Indies.

St. Vincents 12th Augt 1819

My Dear Cousin,

As the Brig Hercules will sail from this Island in a few days for England, I avail myself of the opportunity of sending this letter by her and to inform you that your humble Servant is still in existence. Although I have no News or anything very interesting to tell you, yet I trust you will gratify me by writing, when you can spare a few leisure moments for that purpose, as I have heard nothing from home since I left Winchester. When I last wrote to you how little did I think that the next would be from the West Indies, but it is useless to complain, here we are, and likely to remain for a few Years, not many I hope. I shall give you a slight sketch of our proceedings since we left England, which was on the last day of February and in eight days after that made the Island of Madeira we were becalmed off it for four or five days, and could not get near enough to go into Funchal, after passing the 25th degree of North latitude we caught the trade Winds, which carried us along in a steady manner at the rate of seven or eight knots an hour until we arrived at Barbados on the 3rd of April we remained there about a Week, and as the 4th & 5th Regts arrived at the same time with us, the place became very gay, Dinners and Balls every Day; every Regt. was landed and reviewed, and plenty of inspections made to each. Every Regt has to garrison these Islands except the 25th who remain at Barbados, the 4th have Grenada, Tobago & Trinidad; the 5th Antigua, St. Kitts and Nevis the 9th St. Vincents, St. Lucia & Dominigue; We relieved the 2nd or Queen's Regt at this place, they are gone to Demarara and Balui. The life we lead here is very dull and insipid, although we have received a great deal of civility from the Governor and many of the Planters, but in consequence of the Garrison being situated almost a Mile from the Town, and about six hundred feet above its level we cannot participate in their amusements so frequent as we otherwise would do; and the heat creates such a degree of lassitude, that when I am at any of their Dinner parties I always wish myself back at my own Barrack Rooms. The Day is generally passed in idleness; we have a good Mess and dine at five oClock, generally take a Pint of Madeira after it (which is absolutely necessary here) then retire to one of the Barrack Rooms, to take a flask of Grog, smoke a Cigar and play a rubber or two of Whist, and always in Bed before ten oClock. We have very few white people in these Islands; meet nothing but poor black devils of Negroes and a set of Half and Half Creatures that are as yellow as a Kite's Claw. Everything is very dear and of a very bad quality except what is brought from Europe, even their Fruit is not equal to what I expected except the Pine Apple. Rum is as cheap as Ale in England the Soldiers consequently always drunk, which is the cause of all the Sickness in the West Indies, but I must resume this topic for another letter as I want to enquire after you all. I entreat of you to write to me as soon as you can, and let me know how your good Lady and the Children are, to whom you will make my most kind enquiries, also to your father & Mother and such of Mr. Hutchinson's family as I am acquainted with. With respect to affairs at Mickleton I know no more than the Man in the Moon, doubtless many local occurrences of interest have presented themselves since I last heard from there, you will be good enough to inform them of my having wrote to you and that I never had my health better, which is the only thing they can wish to hear of me; I was very much grieved at my Brother John's misfortune. There is one thing I wish particularly to enquire about, and that is the Exmouth, which I am afraid is off the Road by this time, as every prospector appeared a knavish character especially that Chap Donkin, but of course you will let me know all about, in the mean time believe me to be,

Your ever sincere friend & Cousin,
William Dent.
Assist. Surgn 9th Foot.

Dominica 29th October 1820

My dear Kitt,

Many thanks to you for your obliging letter of the 20th August, which has afforded me the greatest satisfaction to hear you were all in a tolerable state of health; you must tell my Mother that I regret exceedingly that I am unable to transport myself to

Mickleton for a few moments, or else she should not long be tormented with that abominable torture the Toothache. Your letters generally contain some melancholy as well as pleasing intelligence. Poor Joe Fallowfield, I had a peculiar affection for him, as he was as kind and open hearted a School fellow as any I had, but there appears some strong fatality about that family. I feel also for the loss of poor Stephen Shepherd, as he would or ought to have been a guardian to the rest of the family, who I dare say have suffered much from the sudden and unfortunate event. We ought not to speak ill of the dead, but as to Lord Strathmore, I think the very circumstance of his having married that woman marks him as a weak and degraded Man, compared with the rank he held in Society. I must now refer to less melancholy subjects, I see by the Newspapers that the Crops generally have been plentiful, but that you have had too much rain during the Hay Harvest this I hope has not attended the Corn Harvest, and that you have got everything snug housed, I frequently think I could make a good days work myself amongst you if it did not blister my fingers. Your Ideas respecting the purchase Money from Perkins Land, perfectly coincide with mine, I thought £700 would have bought near twice as much; who made the bargain pray; in your next you may mention whether you are making any improvements on it or no. I suppose John is as busy as yourselves in the farming line, how does he manage now as a single Man.

I have now been four months in this Island, and am in a great measure used to the climate without being Sick, as there is always something to be apprehended even in moving from one Island to another, I cannot but think I am very fortunate in keeping my general health good; this Island is the most mountainous in the West Indies and if I were to say in the whole World I would not be much mistaken, like all others it has its good and bad qualities, it suffers from excess of Rain as many of the others do for want of it, Coffee is its principal produce which is of a particular good quality, but on the whole it is considered a very poor Colony.

The part of our Regt stationed here continue very healthy, and if it was not subject to such heavy rains it would be a very pleasant quarter; but the living is bad, fresh meat seldom to be purchased except it is what they call Goat Mutton and that frequently of a very inferior quality. August, September & October are called Hurrican Months, but this Year they have experienced nothing beyond what in England you would call a Gale of Wind, and in fact if you were to see these houses you would not be surprized at their being blown away. I beg you will write to me as often as you can find a little leisure time, as you are the only person in England now with whom I have any correspondence; with my kindest wishes to everyone of the family.

Believe me your very affectionate Brother,
William Dent.

Grenada, 22nd May 1821

My dear Brother,

Your letter of the 20th Feb. I only received three days ago, and find that it has been travelling all over the West Indies. I wrote to my Mother about five Weeks ago, mentioning our change of quarters, and the uncertainty of where I should ultimately be stationed, however that is now settled and I expect to embark almost every day for Trinidad, you will therefore when you again write to me, address at that Island; as soon as I am settled there I will give you every account of it; it is quite close to the Spanish Main, and I understand a very pleasant quarter. With respect to the particulars of your letter I am concerned to find you have had a House of Sickness, however I trust that long before this that your Wife is again returned to her usual good health; I cannot forbear cautioning both you *and* her *of the impropriety of making two at a time, and I am afraid I shall find a House full of Children, the next visit I pay you. I am not surprized, although exceedingly sorry, to hear that my Mother has become so feeble; I dare not say anything against her smoking, for it has now become so habitual that I suppose it would almost destroy her to leave it off; however you may tell her that I hope she makes use of a* cleaner Pipe *than when I last saw her. The description you give of the Lund Hills put me quite in spirits. Don't you think it would make a capital Farm, if we could manage to get a strip of land down to the road, I hope you don't neglect to plant Trees, as I think nothing adds more to the beauty of a Country than its being well wooded. Now for the hunting. You know very well this is a sport that I was always passionately fond of, & after delighting me with the Lund Hills you immediately put me into the fidgets by saying you have established a Subscription Pack of Hounds, the Idea alone of not participating in the amusement makes me quite melancholy, for in this Country if there was ever so much Game, it would be impossible to follow from the excessive heat, But I understand in Trinidad, they have Deer and a species of animal between a Hare & a Rabbit, that affords excellent coursing; they also have Birds of the most beautiful plumage & I shall endeavour to get some of them stuffed to bring to England.*

It is probable we may be three Years longer in this Country, but I believe not more; a Regt. that came out in 1816 is now on its return to England, and we naturally suppose that our stay will not be longer than five years altogether, which is long enough, for the heat is abominable, the Thermometer rises every day to 86° degrees, we have had no Rains for several Months & the Country is burnt to a Cinder. Pray make my respects to the Mr. Olivers who I have no doubt will ultimately overcome all their oppositions; poor Whitcher is put to great shifts; how is Mr. Dixon getting on. Make my kind enquiries to my Father & Mother, John & all friends both at Mickleton & Barnard Castle.

Believe me Yours affectionately,
Wm. Dent.

St. Joseph's Trinidad
7th Oct. 1821

My dear Brother,

I arrived in this Island three Weeks ago after a pleasant passage of two days from Grenada. The Mail from England arrived here last night, I thought probably I might have had the pleasure of hearing from you, but I have not had that gratification. My chief object in writing is to let you know that I am in good health and also of my safe arrival here, for I have no other News which can be at all interesting to you. I joined the Detachment of our Regiment here and find the situation superior to any I have yet seen in the West Indies; the Barracks are situated near to a Village about the size of Middleton, with a fine flat piece of ground in front, a small river also runs near us, which to bathe in is one of the greatest luxuries you can imagine; the Roads here are also excellent, quite level, and nothing but Gigs are made use of by those who can afford them; I have a very good House and generally ride for an hour of two in the Evening. When you write tell me particularly how my Father and Mother are, to whom you will make my most affectionate enquiries as also to John & the whole family. I am also anxious to hear how my Professional friends at Middleton & other places are striving. I am afraid so many will commit great savages on the Community in order to flush themselves into notice. Have you been lately at Barnd. Castle. I have neglected very much not writing to my Cousin Anthy. to whom I am much indebted for his kind hospitality, if you see him tell him so & remember me to his Wife and young ones; What kind of Crops have you had this Summer, and what improvements are you making, you must not neglect giving me a long description of everything. I see by the Newspapers that all has been life and gaiety in England in consequence of the Coronation; but what a melancholy finish the Queen's Death has made, the news of her death arrived before we scarce knew of her being ill. Remember me to all friends and believe me

Your affectionate Brother,
William Dent.

Trinidad, 5th September, 1822

My dear Brother,

I intended to have written to you by the last Packet in answer to your letter which I received by her, but something or other occasioning I have delayed it until the present opportunity. As I observed once before, your letters generally contain some fatal intelligence and I confess my astonishment and regret when I came to read from James Bayles's death, I wish you had entered more fully into a detail of his Sickness, I should like to know how long he was ill and of what disease he died of; as for Rt. Higginson I was not surprized, his time of life and mode of living was sufficient to lead us to expect such an event at no very distant date; To whom has all the property gone, I presume to the younger members of the brother's family. You ask me to give you some account of the Methodist Missioners here; I suppose that part of your letter was dictated by my poor Mother, however I am sorry I cannot give a favourable statement of my attendance or knowing much about them except from hearsay, you must know I am stationed 7 Miles from where they are, their meetings are generally in the evening and in this Country it would not be safe to be exposed to heavy dews at Night, were a Man ever so religiously inclined he would not run this risk long with impunity; we have a Clergyman, who is a Welshman and a very good kind of Man, that performs divine Service to the Troops at this place every second Sunday and everyone is obliged to attend. Has my Cousin A. Harrison arrived in the North yet, and recommenced his Professional duties again. I saw in the Gazette that G. Fielding had purchased his Company in the 23rd I did not think they had so much money to spare; you see everybody gets on in the Service except your humble Servt. and I am afraid you will be thinking me a Stickfast for life; although there are a great many deaths in this Country, it has not fallen on the rank of Surgeons, only one has died since we came to the West Indies; but I have reason to believe, if a casualty should take place that I should be the first for promotion. We have had a long season of Wet this year in the West Indies, nothing but rain and thunder for many weeks past; it has now cleared up a little; it is expected all these Islands will revive again rapidly, in consequence of the new Navigation Laws with America; it will even be a good thing for the Army as we shall get sheep and other articles of life at a much cheaper rate than from England.

You may tell your wife that I shall use every exertion to procure her a collection of Shells, although this Island is not particularly famous for a large size. Poor (   ) how (   ) going on, let me hear something of him (   ) if he is likely to do any good in that hilly country of yours I am happy to find that the two (   ) are in so promising a way, pray remember me to both; also Dixon what has become of him, married and a large family to look after I suppose; I forgot the young parson's name (I don't Mark) still in your neighbourhood. It afforded me much pleasure to hear that my Father & Mother & John were all well, of course you will give my kind enquiries to them, and not forgetting your wife, to every other friend or acquaintance that may enquire after.

Your ever affectionate Brother,
Wm. Dent.

St. Josephs, Trinidad
6th April, 1823

My dear Brother,

I had been anxiously looking out for an Epistle from you, for several Packets past, but had not my anxiety gratified until the last Mail, when I received your letter of the 21st Jany. It afforded me much pleasure to hear you were all well, particularly my Father and Mother; the latter I hope has not fretted much at not hearing from me for so long a period, but it arose from my constant expectation of hearing from you, and an opportunity only offers once a Month for England by Packet. I have enjoyed good health and continue to do so, as well as in any part of the World I ever served in, and I certainly consider myself fortunate, as well as all the Officers of our Regiment since our arrival in the West Indies. I see by the Papers what a very severe Winter you have experienced; Frost and Snow will be quite a treat to me; while you are blowing your fingers, from cold, we are almost burnt to Cinders, from a burning Sun, that causes the Thermometer to rise daily to 85 degrees or upwards. It is confidently reported that we shall be relieved this time twelve months by Regiments from England and Ireland, and if the 9th come to England I shall apply for leave of absence to be amongst you for a couple of Months. You put me quite in the fidgetts when you talk of hunting as you well recollect how passionately fond I always was of that sport and I often think the same is ( ) in the family; but John had always less inclination that way than any of us, and I am rather surprized to hear that he is so keen a houndsman. I heard from Grenada the other day, you know it is the Head Quarters of our Regt, and the

Surgeon has applied for twelve Months leave to go to Ireland, to settle some family affairs, if he should succeed in obtaining leave, I rather think I shall have to replace him, but I shall let you know by the next Packet what arrangement will take place. You complain of the farming business going to the bad; I think there would be no great difficulty in bettering your situation if you would persuade the Government to go to war; that is the only chance of ever surviving the Agricultural interest.

I was sorry to hear of the fate of poor Betty Raine, she was not a very old person; the other two deaths you mention I knew very little of. What improvements have you made about the East end of the Town, I suppose the hedge in front of the house is now able to resist anything, and the Trees are shooting well up, I often picture to myself these little trifles about home. Has John done anything about his place, but his is not as well adapted for improvement as yours; when you write give me a short history of these things, for I assure you it never fails to afford me much pleasure. How are the (   ) friends going on, when you mentioned about hunting, my Uncle Wm. came instantly across my mind, you must make my kind enquiries to them all; is Mary Ann Fallowfield still living there at your home, I hope Anty. Harrison is going on better, but I am afraid I shall not hear from him, in fact I have been more negligent than him, as I promised to write when I last saw him; have they had any more increase of family. Don't forget to pay my best wishes to the Mr. Oliver's, and how happy I am to hear of their success; also Whitham, though he may be considered as an opponent if theirs, still say I enquired after him. I have now to conclude with kind affection to my Father and Mother and every one of our family.

Believe me Your sincere friend and Brother
Willm. Dent.

Trinidad 9th Jany. 1824

My dear Brother Kitt,

Your last kind letter I received about a Month ago, for which I return you many thanks and I am now at a loss how to answer it as I destroyed it immediately after reading it, however I recollect something about a New Road being made to the Westward of you, and I most certainly agree with you that it will be of great advantage to the Country through which it will pass, and I should not be surprized to be sett down at your own door in one of the many Coaches you say are running in that part of the Globe. This letter I know will be considered a very favourable one with you and I know my Mother also, when I tell you that I am no longer Assistant Surgeon in the 9th but a full Surgeon in the 21st Regt. or Royal Scotch Fusiliers, as their Surgeon died, dated 5th Sept. last. It will put me out of the needful, as I have 14s. 1d. (a day).

I have not been well for some time past, although I am much better than I was and I have applied to Head Quarters for leave of absence to come to England for 12 Months, if I should succeed in getting it, you may expect to see me in a few Weeks or Months, but I beg you will not look on it as certain, as I think it very doubtful, at all events you need not write me any more until you hear from me again, or if you do you must address me Mr. Dent Esq., Surgeon 21st Regt. St. Vincent, as the Regt. has lately been removed to there from Demerara, I have not much News to give you as to the state of these Colonies, as now everything is very quiet, we have received two fresh Regts. over from Ireland, the 93rd and the other from old Gibraltar, the 27th which has created a good deal of movement in all the others, but not in the 9th. Should I be fortunate enough to get leave to come home, I have got an Idea into my head that I must take a rib to myself, so look out for a nice, well made lassy for me, that has a little Coin, sufficient to keep herself, and has no objection to a trip to the West Indies. With best regard to all friends.

Believe me
Dear Brother,
Your ever affectionate friend
Wm. Dent. Surgn. 21st Regt. on R.S.F.

Wm. Dent,
Wm. Dent Esq.,
Surgeon 21st Regt.
St. Vincent.

Horse Guards,
9th March 1824

Dear Madam,

I was duly favoured with your letter of the 18th ultimos, enquiring after your Brother in Law Mr. W. Dent, late Asst. Surgeon in the 9th Foot—He was promoted Surgeon to the 21st Regt. 4th Sept. last—We have not received any returns from either of those Regts later than 25th Nov. 1823–At that time Mr. Dent had left the 9th at Grenada, but had not joined the 21st at Demerara—I should have replied to your letter sooner, but have been expecting every day a Mail from the West Indies, bringing Returns of a later date from the 21st Foot, when I hoped to have been able to inform you that he had joined that Corps.

I shall be very happy to forward under a frank, any letters you or his Brothers may wish to write to him, if you will send them to me, & Miss Prattman will inform you of the mode in which they should be enclosed and directed, so that I may receive them free.

I have not heard from New York for a considerable time. My Brother and his family are quite well.

I hope you and your family, with all your other friends, are well—Have the goodness to give my best respects to Mrs. Dawson and Miss Prattman when you see them.—Mr. E. Dawson talks of being (   ) in April.

I am
Dear Madam
Your very obdn. Servant,
C. Jopling.

Addressed to Mrs. Elizabeth Dent, Mickleton.